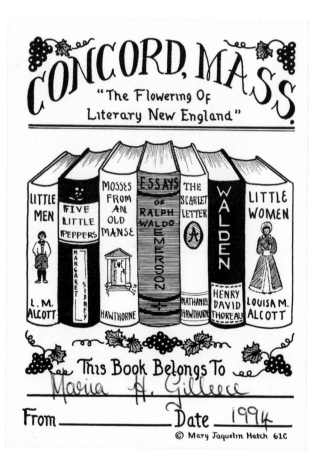

CONCORD, MASS.
"The Flowering Of
Literary New England"

LITTLE MEN — L. M. ALCOTT
FIVE LITTLE PEPPERS — MARGARET SIDNEY
MOSSES FROM AN OLD MANSE — HAWTHORNE
ESSAYS OF RALPH WALDO EMERSON
THE SCARLET LETTER — NATHANIEL HAWTHORNE
WALDEN — HENRY DAVID THOREAU
LITTLE WOMEN — LOUISA M. ALCOTT

This Book Belongs To

Maria H. Gilleece

From _____ Date 1994

© Mary Jaquelin Hatch 61C

LEUKAEMIA

Diagnosis

A Guide to the FAB Classification

A slide Atlas of *Leukaemia Diagnosis, A Guide to the FAB Classification*, based on the contents of this book, is available. In the slide atlas format, the material is split into volumes, each of which is presented in a binder together with numbered 35mm slides of each illustration. Each slide atlas volume also contains a list of abbreviated slide captions for easy reference when using the slides. Further information can be obtained from:

Gower Medical Publishing
Middlesex House
34–42 Cleveland Street
London W1P 5FB

Gower Medical Publishing
101 5th Avenue
New York, NY 10003
USA

Igaku Shoin Ltd
Tokyo International
P.O. Box 5063, Tokyo, Japan

LEUKAEMIA

Diagnosis

A Guide to the FAB Classification

BARBARA J. BAIN

MB BS FRACP MRCPath
Senior Lecturer in Haematology,
St Mary's Hospital Medical School, London, UK

J.B. Lippincott Company PHILADELPHIA
Gower Medical Publishing LONDON · NEW YORK

Distributed in USA and Canada by:
J.B. Lippincott Company
East Washington Square
Philadelphia, PA 19105
USA

Distributed in UK and Continental Europe, Middle East and Africa by:
Harper & Row Ltd
Middlesex House
34–42 Cleveland Street
London W1P 5FB
UK

Distributed in Philippines/Guam and Latin America by:
Harper & Row International
East Washington Square
Philadelphia, PA 19105
USA

Distributed in Australia and New Zealand by:
Harper & Row (Australasia) Pty Ltd
P.O. Box 226
Artarman, N.S.W. 2064
Australia

Distributed in Japan by:
Igaku Shoin Ltd
Tokyo International
P.O. Box 5063
Tokyo
Japan

Distributed in Southeast Asia, Hong Kong, India and Pakistan by:
Harper & Row Publishers (Asia) Pte Ltd
37 Jalan Pemimpin 02–01
Singapore 2057

Project editor:
Zak Knowles

Design:
Balvir Koura

Line artists:
Marion Tasker
Lynda Payne
Lee Smith

British Library Cataloguing in Publication Data:
Bain, Barbara J. (Barbara Jane)
Leukaemia Diagnosis A Guide to the FAB Classification
1. Man. Blood. Leukaemia. Diagnosis.
Laboratory techniques.
I. Title
616.99419075

Library of Congress Cataloging in Publication Data
Bain, Barbara J.
Leukemia diagnosis : a guide to the FAB classification / Barbara J. Bain.
Includes bibliographical references.
1. Leukemia--Classification.   I. Title.
[DNLM: 1. Leukemia--classification.   WH 15 B162L]
RC643.B35   1990
616.99'419'0012--dc20

ISBN: 0-397-44608-X (Lippincott/Gower)

Originated in Hong Kong by Bright Arts

Typesetting by M to N Typesetters, London

Text set in Perpetua; captions and figures set in Gill Sans

Produced by Mandarin Offset. Printed in Hong Kong

PREFACE

Leukaemias are a very heterogeneous group of diseases of varying aetiology, pathogenesis and prognosis. Many systems of classification have been proposed. Among classifications of the acute leukaemias and the related myelodysplastic syndromes, that proposed by a collaborating group of French, American and British haematologists (the FAB group) in 1976 has been widely adopted throughout the world. In this book I have sought to illustrate and explain the FAB classifications and to discuss any ambiguities and consider any problems which arise in applying the classifications. I have discussed immunological markers and cytogenetic abnormalities of leukaemic cells in relation to the FAB classifications and have also dealt in some detail with the related MIC (Morphologic–Immunologic–Cytogenetic) classification. In addition I have discussed the more recently proposed FAB classification of the chronic lymphoid leukaemias and, for completeness, have included a brief chapter on those leukaemias for which the FAB group have not yet proposed a classification.

I have sought to discuss leukaemia diagnosis and classification in a way which will be helpful to trainee haematologists and to laboratory scientists in haematology and in related disciplines and have tried to provide also a useful reference source and teaching aid for practicing haematologists. It is my hope that both haematologists and cytogeneticists will find something of interest and value and each group will learn more of the other's discipline.

B.J.B.

ACKNOWLEDGEMENTS

I would like to express my gratitude to the two British members of the FAB group, Professor David Galton and Professor Daniel Catovsky, who have given me a great deal of help, but at the same time have left me free to express my own opinions. Professor Galton read the entire manuscript and by debating many difficult points with me gave me the benefit of his many years of experience. Professor Catovsky also discussed problem areas and kindly permitted me to photograph blood and bone marrow films from many of his patients. My thanks are also due to Dr Saad Abdalla, Dr Ian Bunce, Dr Sue Fairhead, Dr John Matthews, Dr John Rees, Dr David Swirsky and other colleagues and friends who helped by lending material for photography or by criticizing the manuscript.

CONTENTS

chapter one **ACUTE LEUKAEMIA**

THE NATURE OF LEUKAEMIA

Leukaemia is a neoplastic proliferation of cells of haemopoietic origin which arises following somatic mutation in a single haemopoietic stem cell, the progeny of which form a clone of leukaemic cells. Often a stepwise series of events occur rather than a single genetic alteration. The cell in which the leukaemic transformation occurs may be a lymphoid precursor, a myeloid precursor, or a cell which is capable of differentiating into both lymphoid and myeloid lineages. Myeloid leukaemias may arise in a multipotent stem cell capable of differentiating into cells of erythroid, granulocytic, monocytic and megakaryocytic lineages, or in a lineage-restricted stem cell.

Genetic alterations leading to leukaemic transformation of a cell are often associated with major alterations of chromosomes which can be detected by studying cells of the leukaemic clone in mitosis. Such microscopically detectable abnormalities may give a clue to the site on the chromosome where significant alterations have occurred at a molecular level.

Leukaemias are broadly divided into (i) acute leukaemia which, if untreated, usually causes death in weeks or months and (ii) chronic leukaemia which, if untreated, causes death in months or years.

The clinical manifestations of the leukaemias are due directly or indirectly to the proliferation of leukaemic cells and their infiltration into normal tissues. Increased cell proliferation has metabolic consequences and infiltrating cells also disturb tissue function. Anaemia, neutropenia and thrombocytopenia are important consequences of infiltration of the bone marrow which can lead to infection and haemorrhage.

Lymphoid leukaemias need to be distinguished from lymphomas, which are also neoplastic proliferations of cells of lymphoid origin. Although there is some overlap between the two categories, leukaemias generally have their predominant manifestations in the blood and the bone marrow whilst lymphomas have their predominant manifestations in lymph nodes or other lymphoid tissues.

THE CLASSIFICATION OF ACUTE LEUKAEMIA

The purpose of any pathological classification of disease is to bring together cases which have fundamental biological similarities and which are likely to share features of causation, pathogenesis and natural history. Acute leukaemia comprises a heterogeneous group of conditions which differ in aetiology, pathogenesis, natural history and prognosis. This heterogeneity is reduced if cases of acute leukaemia are divided into acute myeloid leukaemia (AML) and acute lymphoblastic leukaemia (ALL); even then, however, considerable heterogeneity remains within each of the two groups. The recognition of more homogeneous subgroups of biologically similar cases is important as it permits an improved understanding of the leukaemic process and increases the likelihood of causative factors being recognized. Since such subgroups may differ from one another in the cell lineage affected and in their natural history and prognosis, it is likely that the identification of biologically different subgroups will lead ultimately to a different therapeutic approach in some subgroups and to an overall improvement in the prognosis of patients with acute leukaemia.

Although the best criteria for categorizing a case of acute leukaemia as myeloid or lymphoid may be disputed, the importance of such a categorization is beyond doubt. Not only does the natural history differ between the two conditions, but the best current modes of treatment are sufficiently different for an incorrect categorization to adversely affect prognosis. Assigning patients to subtypes of acute myeloid or acute lymphoblastic leukaemia is, at present, less important, but its relevance may increase if some subtypes are found to require a different therapeutic approach. Cases of acute leukaemia may be classified on the basis of morphology, cytochemistry, immunological markers or cytogenetics, or by combinations of these characteristics. Patients may be assigned to the same or different subgroups depending on the characteristics studied and the criteria selected for separating subgroups. All classifications necessarily have an element of arbitrariness, especially when they incorporate continuous variables such as the percentage of cells falling into a defined morphological category, positivity to a certain cytochemical reaction, or the presence of a certain immunological marker.

An ideal classification of acute leukaemia must be biologically relevant. If it is to be useful to the clinical haematologist, as well as to the research scientist, it should also be readily reproducible and easily and widely applicable. Rapid categorization should be possible so that therapeutic decisions can be based on the results of classification. The classification should be widely acceptable and should not change over time so that valid comparisons can be made between different groups of patients. Ideal classifications of acute leukaemia do not yet exist although many have been proposed.

The classification of acute leukaemia now most widely used is that devised by a collaborating group of seven French, American and British haematologists – the French–American–British (FAB) classification[1,2,3,4]. Although various criticisms have been made[5,6] and modifications and expansions have been suggested, it remains the only classification in wide use throughout the world. The FAB group established diagnostic criteria for acute leukaemia as well as proposing a system of classification.

There is usually no difficulty in recognizing that a patient with ALL is in fact suffering from an acute leukaemia, although arbitrary criteria may be necessary to draw a distinction between ALL and the closely related lymphoblastic lymphomas. In the case of AML, more difficulty can arise because of the necessity to distinguish between acute leukaemia and the myelodysplastic syndromes (MDS). The latter term indicates a group of related conditions, characterized by an acquired intrinsic defect in the maturation of myeloid cells, which has been designated myelodysplasia or dysmyelopoiesis. The MDS are clonal disorders which are closely related to, and in some patients may precede, acute leukaemia. In other patients the MDS persist unchanged for many years or lead to death from the complications of bone marrow failure without the development of acute leukaemia; it is therefore justifiable to regard the MDS as diseases in their own right rather than merely as preludes to acute leukaemia. As the prognosis of MDS is generally better than that of acute leukaemia, and because the therapeutic implications are different, it is necessary to make a distinction between acute leukaemia (with or without coexisting myelodysplasia) and a myelodysplastic syndrome in which acute leukaemia has not supervened. The FAB group have defined criteria for distinguishing between acute leukaemia and MDS, and for further categorizing these syndromes. The distinction between AML and MDS will be discussed in this chapter while the further categorization of the MDS will be discussed in Chapter 2.

THE FAB CLASSIFICATION

The FAB classification of acute leukaemia was first published in 1976 following meetings in the preceding two years of a co-operative group set up in the hope of providing a generally acceptable system of classification of this group of diseases[1]. The group hoped thereby to improve accuracy of diagnosis and to standardize classification. The classification was based partly on a scheme proposed by one of the group in collaboration with Sir John Dacie in the preceeding year[7]. The new classification was subsequently expanded, modified and clarified[2,3,4,8]

DIAGNOSING ACUTE LEUKAEMIA

The FAB classification requires that peripheral blood and bone marrow films be examined and that differential counts be performed on both. In the case of bone marrow, a 500-cell differential count is performed. Acute leukaemia is diagnosed if:

(i) at least 30 percent of the total nucleated cells in the bone marrow are blasts, or

(ii) in the case of bone marrow showing erythroid predominance (erythroblasts comprising ≥ 50 percent of total nucleated cells), at least 30 percent of nonerythroid cells are blasts (lymphocytes, plasma cells and macrophages also being excluded from the differential count of nonerythroid cells), or

(iii) if the characteristic morphological features of hypergranular promyelocytic leukaemia (see page 12) are present (Fig. 1.1).

Cases of ALL will all be diagnosed on the first criterion since erythroid hyperplasia does not occur in this condition, but the diagnosis of all cases of AML require application of the second and third criteria. The bone marrow in acute leukaemia is usually hypercellular, or at least normocellular, but this is not necessarily so since some cases of AML meet the criteria for diagnosis when the bone marrow is hypocellular.

DEFINING A BLAST CELL

The enumeration of blasts in the bone marrow is crucial in the diagnosis of acute leukaemia and the definition of a blast is therefore important. Whether immature myeloid cells containing some granules are classified as blasts is a matter of convention. The FAB group have chosen to classify some such cells as myeloblasts rather than as promyelocytes. They recognize two types of myeloblast[8]. Type I blasts lack granules, have uncondensed chromatin, a high nucleocytoplasmic ratio, and usually have prominent nucleoli. Type II blasts resemble Type I blasts except for the presence of a few azurophilic granules and a somewhat lower nucleocytoplasmic ratio. Cells are categorized as promyelocytes rather than as blasts when they develop an eccentric nucleus, a Golgi zone, chromatin condensation (but with retention of a nucleolus), numerous granules and a low nucleocytoplasmic ratio. The cytoplasm, except in the pale Golgi zone, remains basophilic. Cells which have few or no granules, but which show the other characteristics of promyelocytes, are regarded as hypogranular or agranular promyelocytes rather than as blasts. Examples of cells classified as Type II myeloblasts and as promyelocytes are shown in Figs. 1.2 and 1.3. The great majority of lymphoblasts lack granules and are therefore Type I blasts; they resemble Type I myeloblasts but are often

smaller with scanty cytoplasm and may show some chromatin condensation (see Fig. 1.43).

DISTINGUISHING BETWEEN ACUTE MYELOID LEUKAEMIA AND ACUTE LYMPHOBLASTIC LEUKAEMIA

The diagnosis of acute leukaemia therefore requires that blasts (Type I plus Type II) constitute at least 30 percent of either total nucleated cells or nonerythroid cells in the bone marrow. The further classification of acute leukaemia as AML or as ALL is of critical importance. When the FAB classification was first proposed[1], tests to establish the nature of lymphoblasts were not widely available. The group therefore defined as AML cases in which at least 3 percent of the blasts gave positive cytochemical reactions for myeloperoxidase (MPO) or with Sudan Black B (SBB). Cases which appeared to be nonmyeloid were classified as 'lymphoblastic'. The existence of AML cases in which fewer than 3 percent of blasts gave appropriate cytochemical reactions for myeloblasts was not established at that stage, and although a category for cases believed to fall into this group had been included in Dacie and Galton's scheme[7], no such provision was made in the FAB classification. Since 1976 the wider availability and application of immunological markers for B and T lineage lymphoblasts, supplemented by the application of molecular biology techniques to demonstrate rearrangement of immunoglobulin and T-cell receptor genes, has demonstrated that the majority of cases previously classified as 'lymphoblastic' are genuinely lymphoblastic.

However, at the same time, members of the FAB group and others[10,11,12,13] have, by the use of ultrastructural cytochemistry or immunological markers for myeloid cells, shown that a minority of the cases previously categorized as 'lymphoblastic' are in fact acute myeloid leukaemias with minimal maturation*.

Since correct assignment of patients to the categories of AML or ALL is so important for prognosis and for choice of therapy, it is clearly desirable that all cases of apparent lymphoblastic leukaemia should have their nature confirmed by further tests. When lymphoid

---

*In discussing the FAB classification, I have used the terms differentiation and maturation in the sense in which they have been used by the FAB group, that is with differentiation referring to a molecular switch which selects from a multipotential stem cell one pathway or lineage rather than another, and maturation indicating the subsequent changes in the cell and its progeny.

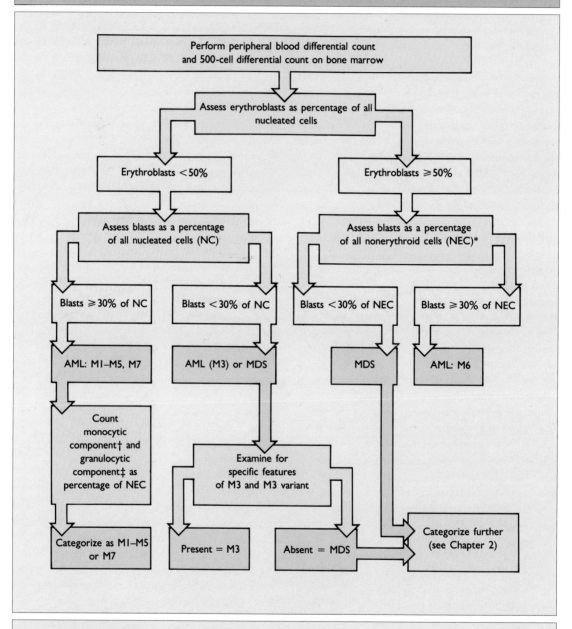

PROCEDURE FOR DIAGNOSING ACUTE MYELOID LEUKAEMIA AND FOR DISTINGUISHING IT FROM MYELODYSPLASTIC SYNDROMES

Perform peripheral blood differential count and 500-cell differential count on bone marrow

Assess erythroblasts as percentage of all nucleated cells

Erythroblasts <50%

Erythroblasts ≥50%

Assess blasts as a percentage of all nucleated cells (NC)

Assess blasts as a percentage of all nonerythroid cells (NEC)*

Blasts ≥30% of NC

Blasts <30% of NC

Blasts <30% of NEC

Blasts ≥30% of NEC

AML: M1–M5, M7

AML (M3) or MDS

MDS

AML: M6

Count monocytic component† and granulocytic component‡ as percentage of NEC

Examine for specific features of M3 and M3 variant

Categorize as M1–M5 or M7

Present = M3

Absent = MDS

Categorize further (see Chapter 2)

* Exclude also lymphocytes, plasma cells, mast cells and macrophages.
† Monoblasts to monocytes.
‡ Myeloblasts to polymorphonuclears.

Fig. 1.1 A procedure for diagnosing acute myeloid leukaemia (AML) and for distinguishing it from the myelodysplastic syndromes (MDS). The criteria in this figure apply to the bone marrow but the blood differential count is required for further categorization. Modifed from Bennett[4] and Bain[9]. See also references 1–3.

markers are negative in 'lymphoblastic' cases, study of myeloid markers is clearly relevant.

Although the large majority of AML cases are recognized by the application of the original criterion of a minimum of 3 percent of blasts being MPO or SBB positive, the following categories which are peroxidase negative by light microscopy need to be recognized as myeloid:

(i) acute myeloblastic leukaemia with minimal evidence of myeloid differentiation;

(ii) some acute monoblastic leukaemias (M5a) with minimal maturation;

(iii) acute leukaemia in which the blast cells have the markers of immature erythroid cells (M6 with minimal maturation);

(iv) acute megakaryoblastic leukaemia (M7))

(v) acute basophilic or mast cell leukaemias without maturation.

It seems desirable that the FAB classification be further expanded to include a category for AML in which there is minimal evidence of myeloid differentiation (see AML M0, page 28).

THE INCIDENCE OF ACUTE LEUKAEMIA

AML has a low incidence in childhood, less than 1 case/ 100,000/year. Among adults the incidence rises increasingly rapidly with age, from approximately 1/100,000/ year in the fourth decade to approximately 10/100,000/

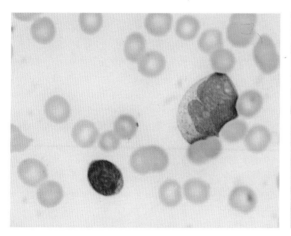

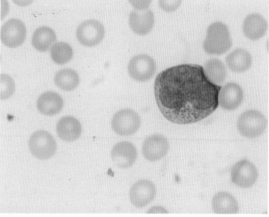

Fig. 1.2 The peripheral blood (PB) film of a patient with AML showing:

(a) a Type II blast with scanty azurophilic granules;

(b) a promyelocyte with more numerous granules and a Golgi zone in the indentation of the nucleus. May–Grünwald–Giemsa (MGG) × 960.

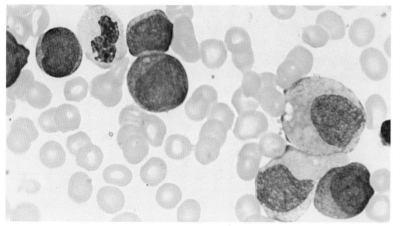

Fig. 1.3 Bone marrow (BM) of a patient with AML [M2/t(8;21)] showing a cell which lacks granules but nevertheless would be classified as a promyelocyte rather than a blast because of its low nucleocytoplasmic ratio; defective granulation of a myelocyte and a neutrophil is also apparent. Type I and Type II blasts are present. MGG × 960.

year in those over 70. ALL is most common in childhood, although cases occur at all ages. In children up to the age of 15 years the overall incidence is of the order of 2.5–3.5/100,000/year; the disease is more common in males than in females and in Whites than in Blacks.

THE CLASSIFICATION OF THE ACUTE MYELOID LEUKAEMIAS

Once criteria for the diagnosis of acute leukaemia have been met and cases have been correctly assigned to the broad categories of myeloid or lymphoid, further classi-fication can be carried out. In the case of AML this categorization is based on a peripheral blood differential count and a 500-cell bone marrow aspirate differential count, supplemented when necessary by cytochemistry, studies of lysozyme levels and more specialized tests. Broadly speaking, acute myeloid leukaemias are divided into acute myeloblastic leukaemia without (M1) and with (M2) maturation, acute hypergranular promyelocytic leukaemia and its variant (M3 and M3V), acute myelomonocytic leukaemia (M4), acute monoblastic (M5a) or monocytic (M5b) leukaemia, acute erythroleukaemia (M6) and acute megakaryoblastic leukaemia (M7).

CRITERIA FOR THE DIAGNOSIS OF ACUTE MYELOID LEUKAEMIA OF M1 SUBTYPE (ACUTE MYELOID LEUKAEMIA WITHOUT MATURATION)[4,8]

Blasts ≥ 90 percent of bone marrow nonerythroid* cells

≥ 3 percent of blasts positive for peroxidase or Sudan Black B

Bone marrow maturing monocytic component (promonocytes to monocytes) ≤ 10 percent of nonerythroid cells

Bone marrow maturing granulocytic component (promyelocytes to polymorphonuclear leucocytes) ≤ 10 percent of nonerythroid cells

* Excludes also lymphocytes, plasma cells, macrophages and mast cells from the count.

Fig. 1.4 Criteria for the diagnosis of AML of M1 subtype.

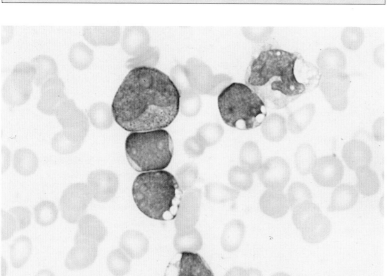

Fig. 1.5 PB film of a patient with M1 AML showing Type I and Type II blasts, some of which are heavily vacuolated, and a promyelocyte. MGG × 960.

Acute myeloblastic leukaemia without maturation – M1

The criteria for the diagnosis of AML M1 are shown in Fig. 1.4 and morphological features are illustrated in Figs. 1.5–1.7. M1 blasts are usually medium to large with a variable nucleocytoplasmic ratio, a round or oval nucleus, one or more nucleoli which range from inconspicuous to prominent, and cytoplasm which sometimes contains Auer rods, a few granules or some vacuoles. Auer rods are crystalline structures thought to be derived from primary granules by coalescence of the granules within autophagic vacuoles. In a minority of cases similar needle-like structures are seen within cytoplasmic vacuoles. In some cases of AML the majority of the blasts are indistinguishable from L2 or even L1 lymphoblasts.

M1 is arbitrarily separated from M2 by having no more than 10 percent of nonerythroid cells consisting of the bone marrow maturing granulocytic component (promyelocytes to polymorphonuclear granulocytes).

The M1 subtype accounts for 15–20 percent of AML cases.

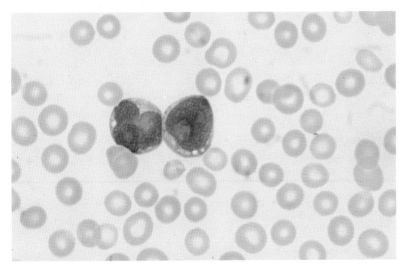

Fig. 1.6 PB film of a patient with M1 AML showing Type I blasts with cytoplasmic vacuolation and nuclear lobulation. MGG × 960.

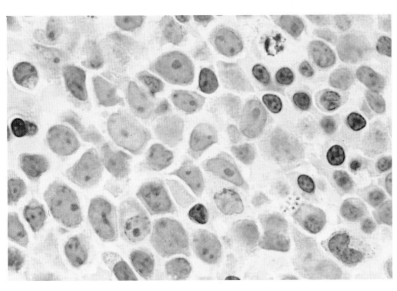

Fig. 1.7 Histological section of a trephine biopsy of a patient with M1 AML. The majority of cells present are blasts with a high nucleocytoplasmic ratio and prominent nucleoli; there are also some erythroblasts and one promyelocyte. Plastic embedded, haematoxylin and eosin (H&E) × 960.

CYTOCHEMICAL REACTIONS IN AML M1

By definition AML M1 has a minimum of 3 percent of blasts being positive for MPO or SBB. Hayhoe and colleagues[14] have found that the SBB reaction is a more sensitive marker of early granulocytic precursors than MPO. M1 blasts are usually also positive for naphthol AS-D chloroacetate esterase (CAE), although this marker is usually less sensitive than either MPO or SBB as an indicator of granulocytic lineage. Myeloblasts give a weak or negative reaction for a number of esterases which are more characteristic of the monocyte lineage, and which are collectively referred to as nonspecific esterases. In the case of α-naphthyl acetate esterase (ANAE) and α-naphthyl butyrate esterase (ANBE) the reaction is usually negative, whereas in the case of naphthol AS-D acetate esterase (NASDA) there is usually a weak fluoride-resistant reaction. Myeloblasts show diffuse acid phosphatase activity which may be weak to strong. The periodic acid-Schiff (PAS) reaction, which identifies a variety of carbohydrates including glycogen, is usually negative, but may show a weak diffuse reaction with superimposed fine granular positivity.

Auer rods give positive reactions for MPO and SBB and occasionally weak PAS reactions. The reaction with CAE is usually weak or negative[14]. Although Auer rods are often detectable on a Romanowsky stain, they are much more numerous and more readily detected on an MPO or SBB stain, and in some cases they are detectable only by the use of such cytochemical stains. Typical cytochemical reactions in a case of M1 AML are shown in Fig. 1.8.

Cases of AML in which the predominant cell is an eosinophiloblast, but where there is no significant maturation, are included in the M1 category. Eosinophiloblasts are positive for MPO and SBB. With the peroxidase stain the granule core may be left unstained. Eosinophiloblasts may be differentiated from myeloblasts committed to the neutrophil lineage by their negative reactions for CAE, and by the demonstration that their peroxidase activity, unlike that of neutrophil lineage blasts, is resistant to cyanide. A combined cytochemical stain for CAE and cyanide-resistant peroxidase is a convenient means of distinguishing between the two lineages[15].

Some cases of acute basophilic leukaemia have sufficient SBB-positive blasts to be categorized as M1. The staining of a basophiloblast with SBB may be metachromatic; whereas the granules of neutrophil and eosinophil lineage blasts show a greenish-black reaction, those of basophiloblasts may be black, grey, pinkish or red.

For further details of cytochemical reactions in leukaemia see Hayhoe and Quaglino[14].

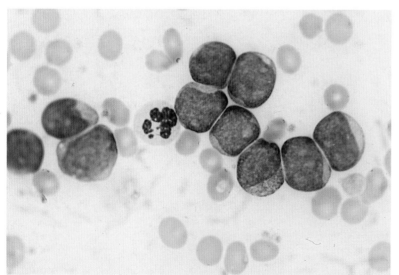

Fig. 1.8 Cytochemical reactions in a patient with M1 AML:

(a) MGG-stained PB film showing largely Type I blasts which in this patient are morphologically similar to lymphoblasts. One leukaemic cell is heavily granulated and would therefore be classified as a promyelocyte; this cell and the presence of a hypogranular neutrophil suggest that the correct diagnosis is M1 AML. MGG × 960.

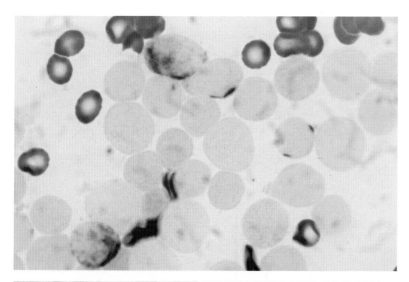

(b) Myeloperoxidase (MPO) stain showing two leukaemic cells with peroxidase-positive granules and two with Auer rods. × 960.

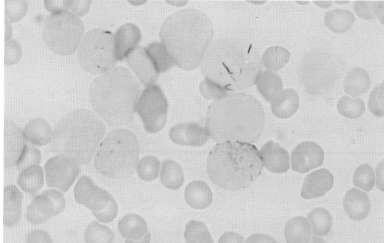

(c) Sudan Black B (SBB) stain of BM showing some blasts with Auer rods and some with granules. × 960.

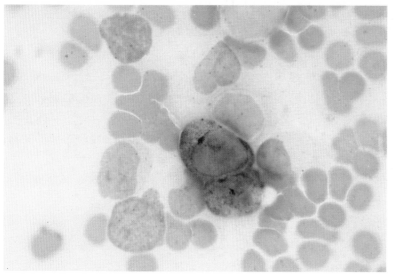

(d) Chloroacetate esterase (CAE) stain of BM showing a positive neutrophil and a positive blast; other blasts present are negative. × 960.

ULTRASTRUCTURAL EXAMINATION IN AML M1

Myeloblasts have a high nucleocytoplasmic ratio, dispersed chromatin and one or more prominent nucleoli. The cytoplasm contains endoplasmic reticulum. Their distinguishing characteristic is the presence of granules. These vary from medium to large in blasts of the neutrophil lineage, and are peroxidase positive on ultrastructural cytochemistry (Fig. 1.9). Eosinophiloblasts contain homogeneous peroxidase-positive granules which may be larger than those of the neutrophil lineage; vacuoles are also common; more mature cells have granules with a crystalline core set in a matrix. In the case of basophiloblasts any of three types of granule may be found[17]:

(i)   large electron-dense granules composed of coarse particles;
(ii) pale granules composed of fine particles;
(iii) theta granules, which are small granules containing pale flocculent material and bisected by a membrane.

PEROXIDASE ACTIVITY OF HAEMOPOIETIC CELLS AS DEMONSTRATED BY ULTRASTRUCTURAL CYTOCHEMISTRY[16,17]				
Cell type	**Myeloblast**	**Basophiloblast/ mast cell precursor**	**Megakaryoblast**	**Proerythroblast**
Site of activity	endoplasmic reticulum, perinuclear space, Golgi zone, granules	granules may or may not be positive; endoplasmic reticulum, perinuclear space and Golgi zone rarely positive	endoplasmic reticulum and perinuclear space only	Golgi zone
Nature of activity	detected by standard technique for MPO* in fixed cells and by PPO** techniques†	more cases are positive by PPO techniques than by MPO technique; activity in ER and perinuclear space detectable	PPO activity is destroyed by fixation in glutaraldehyde so standard MPO technique is negative; PPO detection requires either reaction with DAB prior to fixation*** or a special fixation technique‡	PPO-like activity may be present in Golgi zone

*MPO = myeloperoxidase, Graham and Karnovsky technique[17];

**PPO = platelet peroxidase; ***technique of Roels[17], ‡technique of Breton-Gorius[18].

†Parkin et al.[16] found that a PPO technique‡[18] gave stronger reactions at all sites in the myeloblast than an MPO technique; Polli et al.[17] found that the reaction in membranous structures was stronger by a PPO technique (Roels technique) but the reaction in granules was not.

Fig. 1.9 Peroxidase activity of haemopoietic cells as demonstrated by ultrastructural cytochemistry.

Granules of normal mast cells and their precursors show a scrolled or whorled pattern which is sometimes, but not always, apparent in neoplastic mast cells. Patients with basophil proliferation associated with myeloid leukaemia or myeloproliferative disorders may also have cells with the ultrastructural features of mast cells, and others which have a mixture of granules of basophil and mast cell types. In basophiloblasts and mast-cell precursors the granules may be positive or negative for MPO; the more sensitive platelet peroxidase (PPO) reaction is more often positive (Fig. 1.9). Basophiloblasts can also be identified on ultrastructural cytochemistry by weak staining with ruthenium red[19].

Ultrastructural examination of neutrophil or eosinophil lineage blasts may demonstrate peroxidase-positive Auer rods. They may appear homogeneous, or be composed of longitudinal tubules or dense material with a periodic substructure[20].

Acute myeloblastic leukaemia with maturation – M2

The criteria for the diagnosis of AML M2 are shown in Fig. 1.10. In this context cells included in the granulocytic category are maturing cells from promyelocytes to polymorphonuclear granulocytes, and also cells which differ morphologically from normal promyelocytes but which are too heavily granulated to be classified as blasts. Typical morphological features in M2 AML are illustrated in Figs. 1.11 and 1.12. Maturation of myeloblasts to promyelocytes occurs in both M2 and M3, and promyelocytes are prominent in some cases of M2. Such cases are distinguished from M3 by the lack of hypergranularity

and other specific features of the latter condition (see below). M2 is differentiated from M4 by the monocytic component in the bone marrow being less than 20 percent of nonerythroid cells, and by the lack of other evidence of a major monocytic component (see below). In most cases of M2, granulocytic maturation is along the neutrophil pathway, but maturation to eosinophils or basophils occurs in a minority. Such cases may be designated M2Eo or M2Baso. Other morphologically distinctive categories within M2 are recognized and are characterized by specific cytogenetic abnormalities in addition to typical morphological features (see pages 72 and 78).

The M2 subtype accounts for about 30 percent of AML cases.

CYTOCHEMICAL REACTIONS IN AML M2

The cytochemical reactions of AML M2 are the same as those of M1, but generally reactions are stronger and a higher percentage of cells are positive for MPO and SBB. CAE is more often positive in M2 than in M1, and reactions are stronger. Auer rods are usually more numerous than in M1 and show the same staining reactions. When leukaemic myeloblasts undergo maturation, as in AML M2, there may be a population of neutrophils, presumably derived from the leukaemic blasts, which lack SBB and MPO activity. This may be demonstrated cytochemically or by means of automated differential counters based on the peroxidase reaction which show a low mean peroxidase score and an abnormally placed neutrophil cluster. The neutrophil alkaline phosphatase (NAP) score is also commonly low in M2 AML.

CRITERIA FOR THE DIAGNOSIS OF ACUTE MYELOID LEUKAEMIA OF M2 SUBTYPE (ACUTE MYELOID LEUKAEMIA WITH MATURATION)[4,8]

Blasts 30–89 percent of bone marrow nonerythroid cells

Bone marrow maturing granulocytic component (promyelocytes to polymorphonuclear leucocytes) > 10 percent of nonerythroid cells

Bone marrow monocytic component (monoblasts to monocytes) < 20 percent of nonerythroid cells and other criteria for M4 not met

Fig. 1.10 Criteria for the diagnosis of AML of M2 subtype.

Ultrastructural examination in AML M2 shows blasts with more numerous granules and more frequent Auer rods than in M1; more promyelocytes and maturing granulocytic cells are also present. Mature neutrophils may show a lack of primary, secondary or tertiary granules.

Acute hypergranular promyelocytic leukaemia – M3

In acute hypergranular promyelocytic leukaemia the predominant cell is a highly abnormal promyelocyte and, in the majority of cases, blasts are far below the level of 30

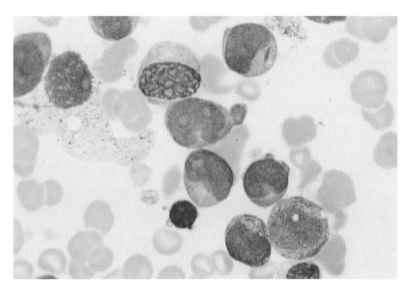

Fig. 1.11 BM film of a patient with M2 AML showing blasts (one of which contains an Auer rod) and a promyelocyte. MGG × 960.

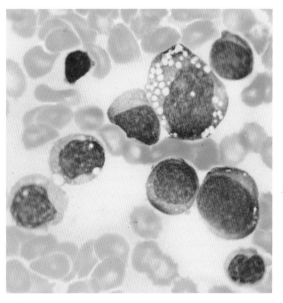

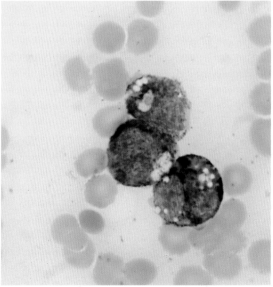

Fig. 1.12 BM film of a patient with M2 AML stained by
(a) MGG;

(b) SBB. In this patient both blasts and maturing cells were heavily vacuolated. × 960.

percent of nucleated bone marrow cells. The distinctive morphology is sufficient to permit a diagnosis and cases are categorized as M3 AML despite the low blast percentage. Abnormalities of coagulation, mainly but not entirely consequent on disseminated intravascular coagulation (DIC), are common in M3 AML. There is also a frequent association with a specific chromosomal translocation, t(15;17).

The morphological features of M3 are shown in Figs. 1.13 and 1.14. The predominant cell is a highly abnormal promyelocyte. This cell has its cytoplasm tightly packed with coarse red or purple granules which may be so dense that the nuclear outline is obscured. Auer rods are present in approaching 50 percent of cases[21]. In some cases there are giant granules or multiple Auer rods which are often in sheafs or 'faggots'. Most cases have a minority of cells which are agranular, have sparse granules, or have fine red or rust-coloured dust-like granules rather than coarse brightly-staining granules. Cells which lack granules, but have lakes of hyaline pink material in the cytoplasm, may also be seen. When the nuclear shape can be discerned, it is found that in the majority of cases some cells have a reniform or folded nucleus, or a bilobed nucleus with only a thin bridge between the two lobes. Dysplastic changes in the erythroid or megakaryocyte lineages do not occur.

Examining an adequate bone marrow aspirate is particularly important in M3 AML as the white cell count is commonly low, and even when there is a leucocytosis typical hypergranular promyelocytes may be rare in the peripheral blood. The specimen may clot during attempted bone marrow aspiration because of the hypercoagulable state, but sufficient cells are usually obtained for diagnosis.

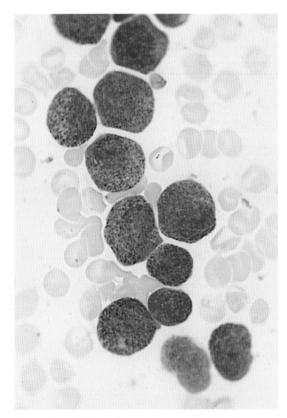

Fig. 1.13 BM film of a patient with M3 AML showing hypergranular promyelocytes, one of which has a giant granule. MGG × 960.

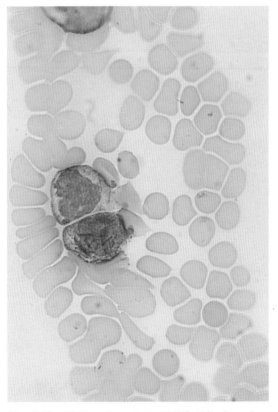

Fig. 1.14 PB film of a patient with M3 AML. One of the abnormal promyelocytes contains loose bundles of Auer rods. MGG × 960.

The variant form of hypergranular promyelocytic leukaemia – M3V

Many years after the description of hypergranular promyelocytic leukaemia it was noted that there were other cases of acute leukaemia which shared with hypergranular promyelocytic leukaemia the characteristic cytogenetic abnormality [t(15;17)][22] and the propensity to DIC, but which had different morphological features. Such cases were recognized as variants of acute hypergranular promyelocytic leukaemia and were designated atypical or microgranular promyelocytic leukaemia[22,23]. Such cases were incorporated into the FAB classification as M3 variant (M3V)[2].

Most cases of M3V are characterized by a cell with a reniform, bilobed, multilobed or convoluted nucleus and either sparse fine granules or agranular cytoplasm (Figs. 1.15 and 1.16). A variable proportion of cells may have multiple Auer rods, fine dust-like granules, or large oval or elliptiform cytoplasmic inclusions with the same staining characteristics as primary granules. Typical hypergranular promyelocytes constitute a small minority of the leukaemic cells in the peripheral blood, but they are usually more numerous in the bone marrow. The white count is usually considerably higher in M3V than in M3.

In a minority of cases of M3V the characteristic cell is a small, abnormal promyelocyte with the same lobulated nucleus as described above but with hyperbasophilic cytoplasm; cytoplasmic projections are sometimes present so that the cell may resemble a megakaryoblast[24]. Such cells are seen in the majority of cases of M3V, but usually as a minor population (Fig. 1.15).

Ultrastructural study shows that in M3V, as in M3, there are many cells in which the cytoplasm is packed with primary granules. There may also be hypogranular cells. In cells with granules, the average granule size is much less than in typical M3; such granules may be below the resolution of the light microscope so that the cell appears agranular, or they may be visualized on light microscopy as fine dust-like granules[22,23,24]. Further evidence that M3 and M3V are correctly categorized together is provided by the observation that the cells of M3V may, in culture, show a marked increase in granularity[25]. Conversely, it has been noted that cases of M3 may show a shift to a lesser degree of hypergranularity on relapse[24].

M3V may be confused with acute monocytic leukaemia (M5b) if blood and bone marrow films are not examined carefully, or if the diagnosis is not considered. When M3 AML appears likely on the basis of the above morphological features, the diagnosis can be confirmed by cytochemistry, ultrastructural examination, immunological markers (see page 68) or, in many cases, by cytogenetic analysis.

The M3 and M3V subtypes together account for 5–10 percent of AML cases.

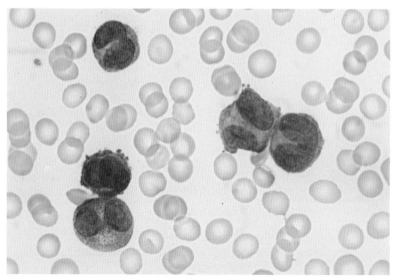

Fig. 1.15 PB film of a patient with M3 variant AML showing cells with bilobed and reniform nuclei and sparse, fine granules. One binucleate cell is present and one cell with basophilic cytoplasm and cytoplasmic projections. MGG × 960.

CYTOCHEMICAL REACTIONS IN AML M3

Hypergranular promyelocytes are usually strongly positive for MPO, SBB and CAE. The PAS reaction usually shows a fine diffuse or dust-like positivity, the reaction being stronger than in M1 and M2. PAS-positive erythroblasts are not generally seen in AML M3. The acid phosphatase reaction is strongly positive. Despite the apparently agranular or hypogranular cells of M3V these cases usually show similar cytochemical reactions to M3[24] (Fig. 1.17); in some cases the reactions are weaker[26]. A potentially confusing cytochemical reaction in both M3 and the variant is the presence in some cases of fluoride-sensitive nonspecific esterase activity[21,23,24], a reactivity otherwise characteristic of monocytic, rather than granulocytic, differentiation. ANAE, ANBE and NASDA may be positive and, as for the monocyte lineage,

the reaction is fluoride sensitive. The reaction is weaker in abnormal promyelocytes than in monocytic cells, and isoenzymes characteristic of the monocyte lineage are not present[26].

Some cells show double staining for nonspecific esterase and CAE. Cases which are positive for ANAE tend to have a weaker reaction for CAE, and occasionally the MPO reaction is also unexpectedly weak[21]. The minority of cases which are positive for nonspecific esterase do not appear to differ from other cases with regard to morphology, haematological parameters, cytogenetic findings or prognosis[21].

Auer rods in M3 are SBB, peroxidase and CAE-positive, and may be weakly PAS positive. On SBB, MPO and CAE staining, the core of the rod may be left unstained and occasionally the core is ANAE positive on a mixed esterase stain[14].

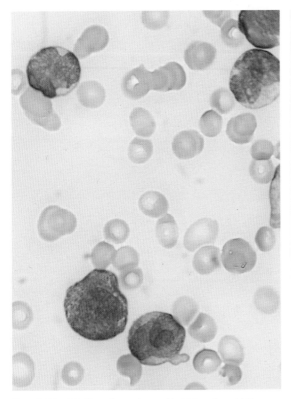 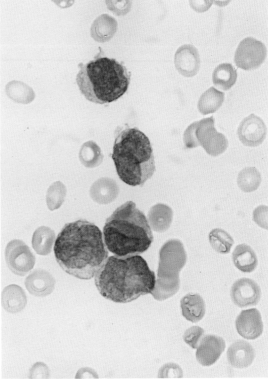

Fig. 1.16 PB film of a patient with M3 variant AML showing:
(a) predominantly agranular cells with twisted nuclei but with one typical hypergranular cell being present;

(b) agranular cells with twisted nuclei; one cell contains a large azurophilic inclusion. MGG × 960.

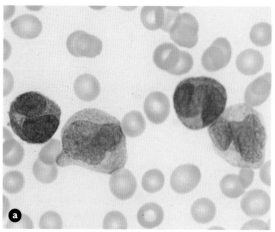

Fig. 1.17 Cytochemical reactions in a patient with M3 variant AML. **(a)** PB and **(b)** BM stained by MGG showing predominantly hypogranular cells with nuclei of characteristic shape. Cytochemical stains of BM show that despite the hypogranularity MPO **(c)**, SBB **(d)**, and CAE **(e)** are strongly positive. × 960.

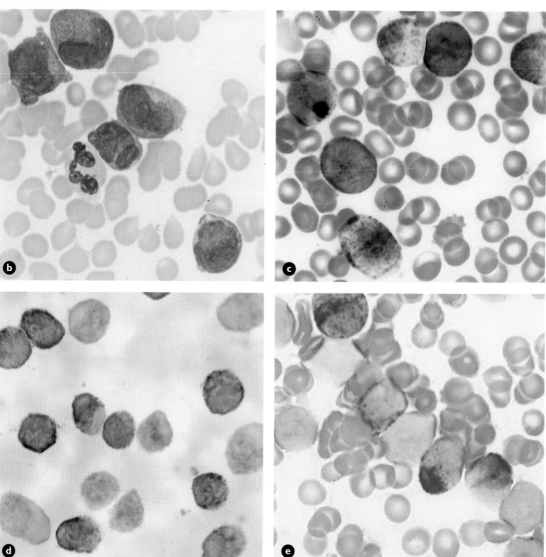

ULTRASTRUCTURAL EXAMINATION IN AML M3

Ultrastructural examination in M3 shows nuclear folding or lobulation. The cytoplasm is packed with numerous granules, which in M3V range from 100–400 nm in diameter and in M3 from 120 to 1000 nm[23,24]. Some cases show Auer rods which differ in structure from those of M1 and M2 AML. They are composed of hexagonal tubular structures[24] and have a different periodicity from other Auer rods. Both granules and Auer rods are peroxidase positive. Some cases show perinuclear microfilaments which otherwise are more characteristic of leukaemia with monocytic differentiation. Grossly dilated endoplasmic reticulum is sometimes seen, particularly in cases with eosinophilic cytoplasm on light microscopy.

Acute myelomonocytic leukaemia – M4

The criteria for the diagnosis of AML of M4 type, that is AML with both granulocytic and monocytic differentiation, or acute myelomonocytic leukaemia, are shown in Fig. 1.18, and typical morphological features in Fig. 1.19.

The criterion for a significant granulocytic component is a morphological one; the granulocytic component, which in this context includes myeloblasts, must be at least 20 percent of bone marrow nonerythroid cells. The presence of a significant monocytic component requires two criteria to be satisfied, which may be both morphological or one morphological and the other cytochemical, as shown in Fig. 1.18. In assessing the monocytic component, in AML M4, monoblasts and promonocytes are included in the count.

Promonocytes are often heavily granulated and can be difficult to distinguish from promyelocytes. The cytochemical criteria for monocytic differentiation are either the presence of fluoride-sensitive naphthol AS-acetate esterase (NASA) or NASDA activity[1], or the presence of ANAE activity[4]. Alternatively, lysozyme activity of leukaemic cells may be demonstrated cytochemically (see Fig. 1.28a), or lysozyme concentration may be measured in serum or urine, an elevation to more than three times the normal value being regarded as significant[4]. Careful examination of the peripheral blood is important if all cases of M4 AML are to be recognized since the bone marrow is sometimes morphologically indistinguishable from that in M2 AML.

CRITERIA FOR THE DIAGNOSIS OF ACUTE MYELOID LEUKAEMIA OF M4 SUBTYPE (ACUTE MYELOMONOCYTIC LEUKAEMIA)[4,8]

Blasts $\geq$ 30 percent of bone marrow nonerythroid cells

Bone marrow granulocytic component (myeloblasts to polymorphonuclear leucocytes) $\geq$ 20 percent of nonerythroid cells

Significant monocytic component as shown by one of the following:

> Bone marrow monocytic component (monoblasts to monocytes) $\geq$ 20 percent of nonerythroid cells and peripheral blood monocytic component $\geq 5 \times 10^9$/l
>
> or
>
> Bone marrow monocytic component (monoblasts to monocytes) $\geq$ 20 percent of nonerythroid cells and confirmed by cytochemistry or increased serum or urinary lysozyme concentration
>
> or
>
> Bone marrow resembling M2 but peripheral blood monocyte component $\geq 5 \times 10^9$/l and confirmed by cytochemistry or increased serum or urinary lysozyme concentration

Fig. 1.18 Criteria for the diagnosis of AML of M4 subtype.

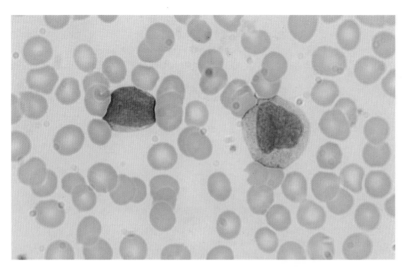

Fig. 1.19 **(a)** PB of a patient with M4 AML showing a myeloblast which is of medium size with a high nucleocytoplasmic ratio, and a monoblast which is larger with more plentiful cytoplasm and a folded nucleus with a lacy chromatin pattern. MGG × 960.

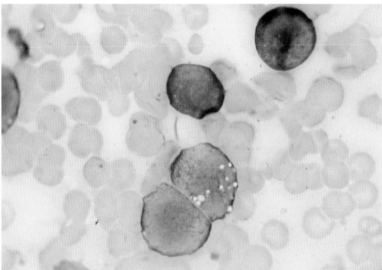

(b) BM of the same patient stained with SBB showing two monoblasts with a weak granular reaction, and two cells of the granulocytic series with a much stronger reaction. × 960.

In AML M4 the granulocytic differentiation is usually along the neutrophil pathway, but it may be eosinophilic (M4Eo), in whole or in part (Fig. 1.20), basophilic (M4 Baso), or both (Fig. 1.21) (see also pages 76 and 78).

The M4 subtype accounts for about 15–20 percent of AML cases.

CYTOCHEMICAL REACTIONS IN AML M4

In M4, some leukaemic cells show cytochemical reactions characteristic of the neutrophil, eosinophil or basophil lineage, and others show reactions typical of the mono-cyte lineage. A double esterase stain for CAE (neutrophil lineage) and ANAE (monocyte lineage)[15] is a convenient method of demonstrating the pattern of differentiation and maturation in M4 (Fig. 1.21c).

ULTRASTRUCTURAL EXAMINATION IN AML M4

Ultrastructural examination shows the findings expected for the granulocyte and monocyte lineages. Eosinophils may show nucleocytoplasmic asynchrony with a mature nucleus, but with only primitive granules lacking a central core[20].

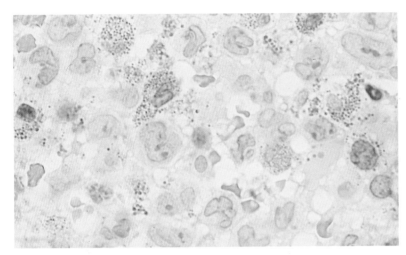

Fig. 1.20 Histological section of a trephine biopsy of a patient with M4Eo AML. Cells are either monoblasts, recognized as large cells with lobulated nuclei containing prominent nucleoli, or eosinophils. Plastic embedded, H&E × 960.

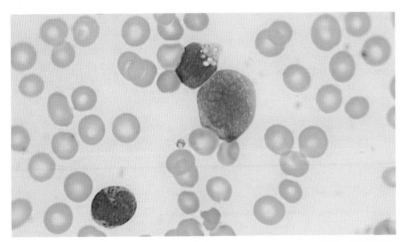

Fig. 1.21 PB film of a patient with M4 AML [M4Eo/inv(16)] who had both eosinophil and basophil differentiation:

(a) a blast cell and two primitive cells containing basophil granules; one of the latter is vacuolated. MGG × 960.

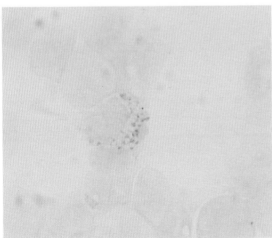

(b) toluidine blue stain showing metachromatic staining of a basophil precursor. × 960.

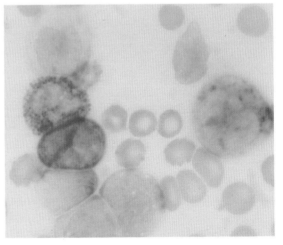

(c) double esterase stain showing positivity of the granulocyte series with CAE (red) and positivity of the monocyte series with α-naphthyl acetate (nonspecific) esterase (brownish-black). × 960.

Acute monocytic/monoblastic leukaemia – M5

The criteria for the diagnosis of acute monocytic/monoblastic leukaemia, AML M5, are shown in Fig. 1.22, and typical morphological features in Figs. 1.23–1.26. M5 is further divided into M5a (acute monoblastic leukaemia) and M5b (acute monocytic leukaemia) on the basis of whether monoblasts comprise at least 80 percent of the total bone marrow monocytic component. Monoblasts are large cells with plentiful cytoplasm which is sometimes vacuolated, and is usually moderately, occasionally strongly, basophilic; scattered fine azurophilic granules may be present. The nucleus varies from round (in the most primitive monoblasts) to convoluted with a delicate chromatin pattern and one or several nucleoli, which are often large and prominent. Promonocytes have prominent azurophilic granules and cytoplasm which is usually more basophilic than that of monoblasts. Monocytes have a lower nucleocytoplasmic ratio, a lobulated nucleus and weakly basophilic, often vacuolated, cytoplasm with an irregular outline. In monocytic leukaemias there is often disorderly maturation producing nucleocytoplasmic asynchrony and dysplastic cells; this can make it difficult to classify cells reliably as monoblasts, promonocytes or monocytes. The peripheral blood may show cells of monocytic lineage which are more mature than those present in the bone marrow (Fig. 1.25). Monoblast/monocyte differentiation may be confirmed by cytochemistry, by measurement of serum or urinary lysozyme levels, or by ultrastructural examination.

The M5 subtype accounts for about 15 percent of AML cases.

CRITERIA FOR THE DIAGNOSIS OF ACUTE MYELOID LEUKAEMIA OF M5 SUBTYPE (ACUTE MONOBLASTIC/ MONOCYTIC LEUKAEMIA)[4,8]	
Blasts ⩾ 30 percent of bone marrow nonerythroid cells	
Bone marrow monocytic component ⩾ 80 percent of nonerythroid cells	
Acute monoblastic leukaemia (M5a)	Acute monocytic leukaemia (M5b)
Monoblasts ⩾ 80 percent of bone marrow monocytic component	Monoblasts < 80 percent of bone marrow monocytic component

Fig. 1.22 Criteria for the diagnosis of AML of M5 subtype.

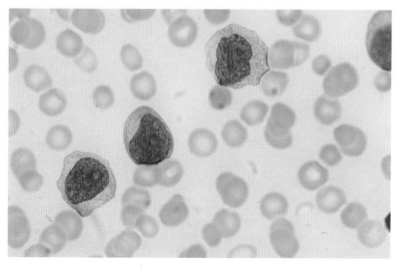

Fig. 1.23 PB film of a patient with M5a AML showing three monoblasts. MGG × 960.

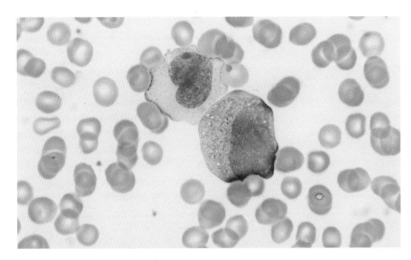

Fig. 1.24 PB of a patient with M5b AML showing a monocyte and a promonocyte; the latter is moderately heavily granulated. MGG × 960.

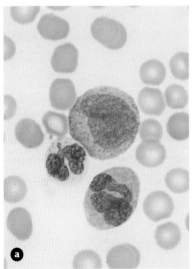
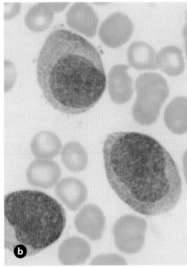

Fig. 1.25 PB and BM of a patient with M5b AML in whom the PB cells were more mature than the BM cells.
(a) PB showing a promonocyte and a monocyte with a nucleus of abnormal shape; the third cell is probably an abnormal neutrophil. MGG × 960.
(b) BM showing predominantly monoblasts and promonocytes. MGG × 960.

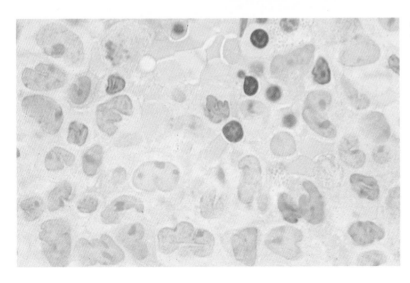

Fig. 1.26 Histological section of trephine biopsy of a patient with M5b AML and myelodysplasia. Monoblasts and monocytes can be identified; the former are the larger cells with a round or lobulated nucleus, a dispersed chromatin pattern and prominent nucleoli, whereas the latter are smaller with lobulated nuclei and more chromatin clumping. The cells with smaller dark nuclei are erythroblasts, one of which has a nucleus of abnormal shape. H&E × 960.

CYTOCHEMICAL REACTIONS IN AML M5

In acute monoblastic leukaemia (M5a), MPO and SBB reactions are commonly negative, although a scattered fine granular positivity may be present. CAE is negative or very weak. Hayhoe and colleagues[14] found SBB to be more sensitive than MPO in the detection of monoblasts, and noted that with SBB, monoblasts usually showed scattered fine granules, whereas in myeloblasts the reaction was strong and was either localized or filled the whole cell. With MPO, monoblasts were found to be characteristically negative. Monoblasts are strongly positive for ANAE (Fig. 1.27a), ANBE, NASA (Fig. 1.27b, c) and NASDA (nonspecific esterases). All these esterase activities are inhibited by fluoride, but only in the case of NASA and NASDA is it necessary to do the test with and without fluoride to convey specificity; in the case of ANAE and ANBE the reaction is negative or weak in cells of the granulocytic lineage. Aberrant esterase reactions are sometimes seen; occasional cases have negative reactions for nonspecific esterases, or give positive reactions for both chloroacetate and nonspecific esterases. Monoblasts show a diffuse positivity for acid phosphatase which, along with nonspecific esterase activity, appears in advance of MPO and SBB positivity. Lysozyme activity, which appears at about the same time as MPO activity, may be demonstrated cytochemically (Fig. 1.28a). The PAS reaction of monoblasts is either negative, or diffusely positive with a superimposed fine or coarse granular positivity or, occasionally, superimposed PAS-positive

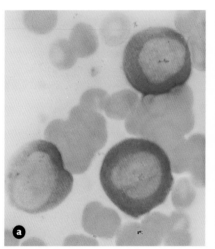
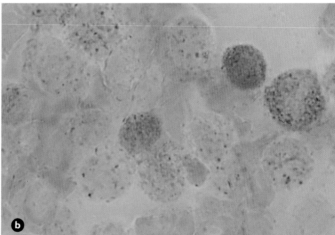
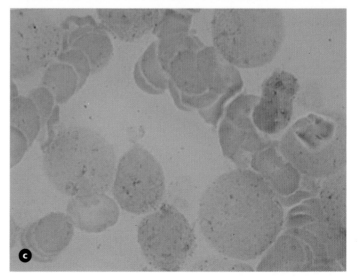

Fig. 1.27 **(a)** BM of a patient with M5a AML stained for α-naphthyl acetate (nonspecific) esterase activity. × 960. **(b, c)** BM of a patient with M5b AML stained for naphthol AS acetate esterase (NASA) activity **(b)** without and **(c)** with fluoride; inhibition of activity by fluoride is apparent. × 960.

blocks (Fig. 1.28b). In M5 the NAP score is normal or high, in contrast to the low score which may be seen in cases of AML where abnormal granulocytic maturation is occurring.

ULTRASTRUCTURAL EXAMINATION IN AML M5

Monoblasts are larger than myeloblasts with more voluminous cytoplasm, which may be vacuolated or show pseudopodial projections. The nucleus is round, lobulated or twisted with a characteristically large nucleolus. Perinuclear bundles of microfilaments may be present. Monoblasts may contain granules which are smaller than those of myeloblasts. The earliest granule to appear is a very small peripherally-situated granule which

is negative for MPO but positive for acid phosphatase[27]. The latter activity may also be present in the Golgi apparatus. The earliest monoblasts are completely MPO negative. MPO positivity is first detected in the perinuclear envelope, Golgi apparatus and endoplasmic reticulum. Subsequently, MPO-positive granules appear; they are smaller than the MPO-positive granules of the neutrophil lineage and may sometimes be detectable when MPO is negative by light microscopy. When the first peroxidase-positive granules appear some chromatin condensation is already occurring and some authors prefer to classify these cells as promonocytes. The PPO technique is more sensitive to peroxidase activity in the monocyte lineage than the MPO technique. Nonspecific esterase activity can also be detected at ultrastructural level.

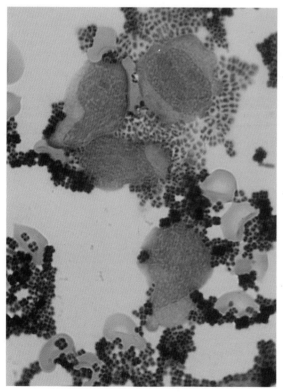

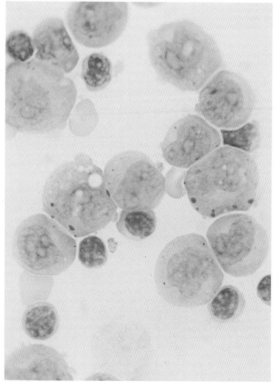

Fig. 1.28 **(a)** Lysozyme preparation from a patient with M5b AML. Leukaemic cells have been mixed with a suspension of *Micrococcus lysodeikticus* bacteria; some of the leukaemic cells have secreted lysozyme which has lysed adjacent bacteria, which appear paler in comparison with intact bacteria (same patient as Fig. 1.27b, c). MGG × 960.

(b) Periodic acid-Schiff (PAS) stain of a PB cytospin preparation from a patient with M5a AML showing block-positivity superimposed on fine granular and diffuse positivity. × 960.

Acute myeloid leukaemia with predominant erythroid differentiation – M6

The criteria for the diagnosis of M6, or AML with predominant erythroid differentiation, are shown in Fig. 1.29, and morphological features are shown in Figs. 1.30–1.33. M6 may be regarded as the erythroleukaemic transformation of MDS, with the cut-off point between the two being arbitrary. Moderate to marked erythroid dysplasia is common, with erythroid precursors showing features such as nucleocytoplasmic asynchrony, nuclear lobulation, karyorrhexis, binuclearity and cytoplasmic vacuolation. In some cases, giant and multinucleated erythroid cells are prominent. Erythropoiesis may be predominantly megaloblastic. Phagocytosis, particularly erythrophagocytosis, by abnormal erythroid precursors is not uncommon. The nonerythroid component in M6 may resemble any of the other FAB categories with the exception of M3. Myeloblasts may show Auer rods, and the granulocytic lineage and megakaryocytes commonly show dysplastic features.

FAB criteria for M6 require that at least 50 percent of bone marrow nucleated cells are recognizable erythroblasts, and that at least 30 percent of the nonerythroid cells are blasts. There are other cases of AML in which the leukaemic cells appear by light microscopy to be undifferentiated blasts, but which can be shown by immunological markers or ultrastructural examination to be very primitive erythroid cells. It seems desirable that these cases (which are rare except when AML occurs in Down's syndrome patients)[28] should be classified as M6.

Overall, the M6 subtype accounts for about 3–4 percent of AML cases.

CRITERIA FOR THE DIAGNOSIS OF ACUTE MYELOID LEUKAEMIA OF M6 SUBTYPE (ACUTE ERYTHROLEUKAEMIA)[4,8]
Erythroblasts ≥ 50 percent of bone marrow nucleated cells
Blasts ≥ 30 percent of bone marrow nonerythroid cells

Fig. 1.29 Criteria for the diagnosis of AML of M6 subtype.

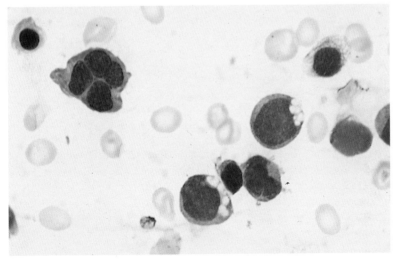

Fig. 1.30 BM film from a patient with M6 AML (erythroleukaemia) showing a multinucleated erythroblast and two heavily vacuolated myeloblasts. MGG × 960.

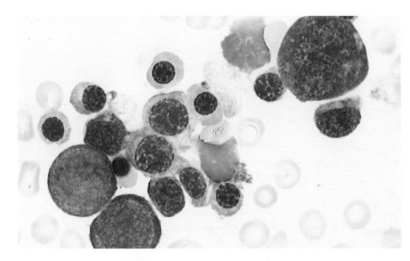

Fig. 1.31 BM film from a patient with M6 AML showing marked erythroid hyperplasia but only mild dyserythropoiesis; one binucleated erythroblast is present. MGG × 960.

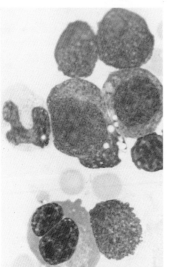
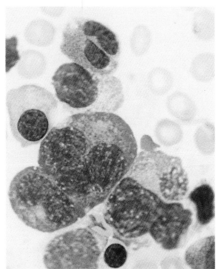

Fig. 1.32 BM film from a patient with M6 AML showing: a binucleated erythroblast and two vacuolated erythroblasts (left); a giant multinucleated erythroblast (right). MGG × 960.

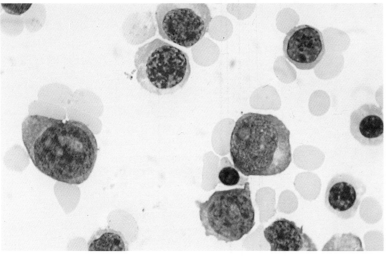

Fig. 1.33 A cytospin preparation of BM cells of a patient with M6 AML showing late erythroblasts and three undifferentiated blasts. A positive reaction of the blast cells with a monoclonal antibody (McAb) to glycophorin A showed that these were primitive erythroid cells. MGG × 960.

CYTOCHEMICAL REACTIONS IN AML M6

In M6, myeloblasts and any Auer rods show the same cytochemical reactions as in other categories of myeloid leukaemia. The NAP score may be reduced or increased, and a population of neutrophils lacking SBB and MPO activity may be present.

On a PAS stain, the erythroblasts show diffuse or finely granular positivity with or without superimposed coarse granular or block positivity. Hayhoe and colleagues[14] have described a characteristic block or granular positivity in early cells, and diffuse positivity in late erythroblasts and some erythrocytes. PAS positivity is not pathognomonic of erythroleukaemia, being seen also in MDS and in iron deficiency anaemia, severe haemolytic anaemia, thalassaemia major and in occasional cases of megaloblastic anaemia. PAS positivity of erythroblasts may also be seen in other categories of AML, and in this case may well indicate that the erythroblasts, despite being less than 50 percent of nucleated cells, are part of the leukaemic clone. Erythroblasts in M6 may have acid phosphatase activity which is localized to the Golgi zone[17]; they are usually positive for ANAE and ANBE[14]. These reactions differentiate them from the erythroblasts of congenital dyserythropoietic anaemia, in which acid phosphatase and nonspecific esterase reactions are negative, but positive reactions can also be seen in megaloblastic erythropoiesis consequent on pernicious anaemia[14]. A Perls' stain for iron may show coarse siderotic granules; in a minority of cases numerous ring sideroblasts are present.

ULTRASTRUCTURAL EXAMINATION IN AML M6

Primitive erythroblasts have a round nucleus, a well-defined nucleolus, minimal chromatin condensation, numerous polyribosomes, long strands of endoplasmic reticulum, numerous mitochondria and an active Golgi apparatus. Surface vesicles and invaginations are common. Clusters of granules which are acid phosphatase positive may be present close to the Golgi apparatus. Primitive cells can be positively identified as erythroid by the presence in the cytoplasm of aggregates of ferritin molecules or iron-laden mitochondria, or by the presence of rhopheocytosis (invagination of the cell membrane in association with extracellular ferritin molecules). Ultrastructural cytochemistry shows negative reactions for MPO, but PPO-like activity has been described in the Golgi zone.

Acute megakaryoblastic leukaemia – M7

Acute megakaryoblastic leukaemia was not included in the original FAB classification, but following the demonstration that some apparently undifferentiated blasts were actually megakaryoblasts this category was added[3] (Fig. 1.34). Leukaemic megakaryoblasts are commonly highly polymorphic. Prominent and multiple nucleoli and cytoplasmic basophilia have been noted[17]. In some cases the diagnosis can be suspected from the morphology when blasts show cytoplasmic protrusions or budding of platelets, or when blasts coexist with apparently bare nuclei, with large bizarre platelets, or with a population of more mature cells showing megakaryocyte differentiation. In other cases either the blasts cannot be distinguished from myeloblasts or they resemble lymphoblasts, being small with a very high nucleocytoplasmic ratio and with some chromatin condensation. The nature of megakaryoblasts may be suggested by the pattern of cytochemical reactions; they can be positively identified by ultrastructural examination (see below) or by immunological techniques which demonstrate positive reactions for factor VIII-related antigen, platelet factor 4, platelet-derived growth factor, or platelet membrane glycoproteins (see page 68). Morphological features in cases of M7 AML are shown in Figs. 1.35 and 1.36

The M7 subtype accounts for 2–4 percent of AML cases.

CYTOCHEMICAL REACTIONS IN AML M7

Megakaryoblasts give negative reactions for MPO, SBB and CAE. The more mature cells of this lineage are PAS positive and have fluoride-sensitive nonspecific esterase activity. On PAS staining there are positive granules on a

---

CRITERIA FOR THE DIAGNOSIS OF ACUTE MYELOID LEUKAEMIA OF M7 SUBTYPE (ACUTE MEGAKARYOBLASTIC LEUKAEMIA)[3]

Blasts ≥ 30 percent of bone marrow nucleated cells

Blasts demonstrated to be megakaryoblasts by immunological markers, ultrastructural morphology or ultrastructural cytochemistry

Fig. 1.34 Criteria for the diagnosis of AML of M7 subtype.

diffusely positive background. In some cases, the positive granules are peripheral or are packed into the cytoplasmic blebs. The nonspecific esterase activity is best demonstrated by ANAE activity which gives weak to strong reactions, whereas ANBE gives negative or weak reactions; this pattern differs from the esterase activity of the monocyte lineage where ANAE and ANBE activities are equally strong. Esterase activity is often localized to the Golgi zone[17]. There is a similar localization of acid phosphatase activity which is tartrate sensitive[17]. When the leukaemic cells are very immature, PAS and nonspecific esterase reactions are negative.

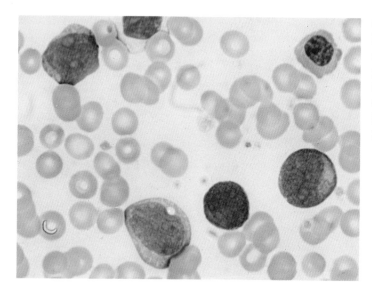

Fig. 1.35 PB film from a patient with Down's syndrome with M7 AML (acute megakaryoblastic leukaemia); blasts are pleomorphic with no specific distinguishing features. The nature of the leukaemia was demonstrated by a positive reaction with a McAb to platelet glycoprotein IIb/IIIa. MGG × 960.

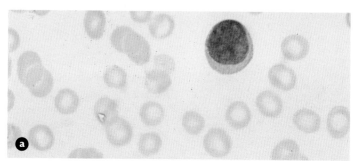

Fig. 1.36 PB and BM films from a patient with M7 AML presenting as acute myelofibrosis; the nature of the leukaemia was demonstrated by a positive reaction for platelet peroxidase:
(a) PB showing mild anisocytosis and a blast cell with no distinguishing features;

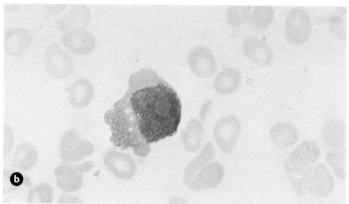

(b) BM showing megakaryoblast. MGG × 960.

ULTRASTRUCTURAL EXAMINATION IN AML M7

On ultrastructural examination some megakaryoblasts resemble lymphoblasts, being small with a high nucleo-cytoplasmic ratio and no distinguishing features. More mature cells are larger and may have α-granules, bull's-eye granules or demarcation membranes[17,29]. On ultrastructural cytochemistry, megakaryoblasts show peroxidase activity which is confined to the endoplasmic reticulum and perinuclear space, and is detectable only by the PPO reaction[30,31] (Fig. 1.9).

Acute myeloid leukaemia with minimal evidence of myeloid differentiation – M0

The FAB classification, as published in 1976[1], assigned to the 'lymphoblastic' category all cases which did not have at least minimal cytochemical evidence of myeloid differentiation. As discussed on page 3, it now seems more appropriate to reassign to an M0 (M nought or M zero) category (Fig. 1.37) those cases which lack lymphoid markers and in which further tests show minimal evidence of myeloid differentiation. Acceptable

CRITERIA FOR THE DIAGNOSIS OF ACUTE MYELOID LEUKAEMIA OF M0 SUBTYPE (AML WITH MINIMAL EVIDENCE OF MYELOID DIFFERENTIATION)

Blasts ≥ 30 percent of bone marrow nucleated cells

< 3 percent of blasts positive for Sudan Black B or for peroxidase by light microscopy

Blasts demonstrated to be myeloblasts by immunological markers or by ultrastructural cytochemistry

Fig. 1.37 Criteria for the diagnosis of AML of M0 subtype.

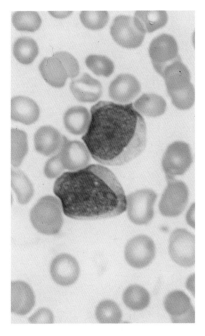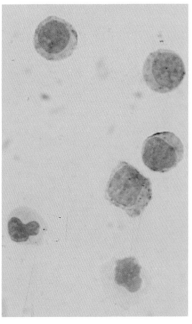

Fig. 1.38 MGG-stained PB film from a patient with M0 AML showing two blasts (left); cytospin preparation of PB mononuclear cells stained by an immunoperoxidase technique with the McAb MCS.2 (CD13) which is specific for myeloid cells (right). Blasts are positive whereas two lymphocytes are negative. × 960.

criteria for such differentiation include:

(i) demonstration of MPO activity by ultrastructural cytochemistry[12] (Fig. 1.9);
(ii) demonstration of MPO protein by use of a monoclonal antibody which recognizes its antigenic activity[13];
(iii) demonstration of other myeloid antigens by the use of monoclonal antibodies such as those belonging to the CD13 and CD33 clusters which appear to be specific for myeloid cells[12,13];
(iv) demonstration of the cytochemical reactions (see below) or ultrastructural features (see page 10) of basophiloblasts (M0Baso).

In investigating cases of apparently undifferentiated acute leukaemia, the differential diagnosis should include not only M0 but also M7 and M6 with minimal maturation. Only cases positively identified as myeloid should be categorized as M0. The very small number of cases which cannot be demonstrated to be either lymphoid or myeloid should be categorized as 'undifferentiated' or 'unclassifiable' (although a clinician treating such a patient will necessarily have to make a decision as to whether treatment suitable for ALL or AML is more appropriate in a specific case). Typical examples of M0 AML are shown in Figs. 1.38–40.

Cases of AML M0 and M1 are much more likely to be positive for terminal deoxynucleotidyl transferase (TdT) than cases showing more evidence of maturation (M2 to M5); M6 and M7 are characteristically TdT negative[12].

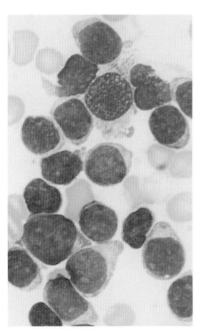
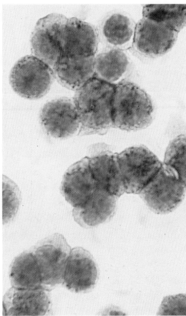

Fig. 1.39 PB and BM preparations from a patient with M0 AML: BM film stained by MGG showing agranular blasts (left); immunoperoxidase reaction of PB cells with the McAb MCS.2 (CD13) showing many strongly positive blasts; the blasts were also positive for the Ia antigen and terminal deoxynucleotidyl transferase (TdT) and with the McAb 3C5 (CD34) (right). × 960.

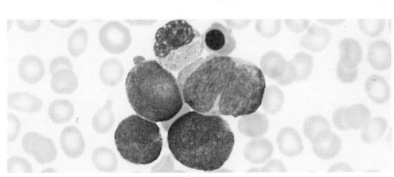

Fig. 1.40 BM film of a patient with M0 AML showing agranular pleomorphic blasts with a high nucleocytoplasmic ratio; the presence of a neutrophil with a nucleus of abnormal shape suggests the correct diagnosis. MGG × 960.

CYTOCHEMICAL REACTIONS IN AML M0

By definition less than 3 percent of the blasts in AML M0 are positive for MPO, SBB or CAE, since such positivity would lead to the case being classified as M1. Similarly, blasts are negative for the nonspecific esterases or the case would be categorized as M5.

In acute basophilic leukaemia[19], SBB is commonly negative and MPO is negative by light microscopy. Often CAE is also negative, although it is weakly positive in later cells of the basophil lineage. Such cases do not meet the criteria for M1 and should be categorized as M0. (Other cases of acute basophilic leukaemia will fall into M1, M2 or M4 categories.) When a basophilic or mast cell leukaemia is suspected, the nature of the blasts can be confirmed by metachromatic staining with toluidine blue or Astra blue. The PAS stain shows positive blocks, or elongated or irregular lakes.

ULTRASTRUCTURAL EXAMINATION IN AML M0

Ultrastructural cytochemistry is a sensitive means of identifying AML M0. The characteristic findings in myeloblasts committed to the neutrophil or basophil lineages are discussed on page 10, and the expected results of ultrastructural cytochemistry are shown in Fig. 1.9.

CLINICAL CORRELATES OF ACUTE MYELOID LEUKAEMIA FAB CATEGORIES

Certain clinical and haematological features correlate with the FAB classes, although such correlations are closer if cytogenetic abnormalities are considered in addition to FAB class (see Chapter 3).

Patients with M3 AML are younger than average, usually have DIC, and often have a relatively low white cell count. M3 does not demonstrate a preleukaemic myelodysplastic phase and rarely, if ever, occurs as a secondary leukaemia following radiotherapy/chemotherapy. Patients with M3V tend to have higher white cell counts but otherwise show features similar to those of typical M3. Patients with M5 often have gum hypertrophy and skin infiltration, and this is true to a lesser extent of M4. Hepatomegaly, splenomegaly and lymphadenopathy are also most common in M5. Both M4 and M5 may have serous effusions in joints and in the pericardium, and the risk of CNS leukaemia (both leptomeningeal and intracerebral) has been reported to be highest in these categories. M7 commonly presents with pancytopenia and with the clinical features of acute myelofibrosis[17,31]. M6[28] and M7 are overrepresented among cases of AML in infants with Down's syndrome.

The FAB category correlates with prognosis, although not strongly. In a study of 716 patients with AML the prognostic factors in order of significance were age, platelet count, FAB category, the presence of DIC, the percentage of myeloblasts in the peripheral blood and whether the leukaemia was secondary or *de novo*[32]. The FAB category with the best prognosis was M2, followed in order by M4, M1, M3 plus M3V, M5 and M6. When analysis was confined to 291 optimally treated patients the FAB category remained significant, with the prognostic factors in order of significance being age, platelet count, percentage of peripheral blood myeloblasts and the FAB category. In other published studies there has also been overall a higher remission rate in M2 and M4 than in M1, with M5 and M6 showing the lowest remission rates. Reports of the treatment outcome in small numbers of M0 patients suggest that they have a worse prognosis than all other categories of AML[10]. Prognostic differences are greater if patients are further categorized by means of cytogenetic analysis, in addition to the FAB classification.

The FAB category as yet has little influence on the treatment given to a patient with AML, although the recognition of M3 and M3V is important in alerting the clinician to the likelihood of DIC and the need to give appropriate treatment for this. It is likely, however, that more detailed classification of patients using cytogenetic findings, in addition to the FAB category, will soon lead to the use of different treatment protocols in various subgroups of patients.

THE CLASSIFICATION OF ACUTE LYMPHOBLASTIC LEUKAEMIA

Acute lymphoblastic leukaemia can be diagnosed from a combination of morphological features and cytochemical reactions[1]; tests for enzymes characteristic of myeloid cells are negative, whereas the PAS reaction often shows a distinctive pattern (see below). When facilities are available it is desirable that cases of apparent ALL should be further investigated by immunological markers for T- and B-lineage lymphoblasts in order to confirm the diagnosis. The immunological categorization of ALL is discussed in detail in Chapter 3 and is summarized in Figs. 3.4 and 3.5. It is sufficient at this stage to say that B-lineage ALL includes a small minority of cases with the markers of mature B cells (B-ALL), and among the majority population of B-cell precursor ALL there is a major subgroup of cases designated common ALL (cALL). Cases of ALL can also be categorized morphologically

into three subgroups – L1, L2 and L3 (Fig. 1.41) – but apart from a strong correlation between B-ALL and L3 morphology there is no clear relationship between the FAB morphological category and the immunological classification.

The recognition of cases of L3 ALL is generally straight-forward, but the categorization of a case as L1 or L2 is

MORPHOLOGICAL FEATURES OF ALL SUBTYPES

	L1	L2	L3
Cell size	Mainly small	Large, heterogeneous	Large, homogeneous
Nuclear chromatin	fairly homogeneous	heterogeneous	finely stippled; homogeneous
Nuclear shape	mainly regular	irregular; clefting and indentation common	regular; oval to round
Nucleolus	not visible or small and inconspicuous	usually visible; often large	usually prominent
Cytoplasm	scanty	variable; often abundant	moderately abundant
Cytoplasmic basophilia	slight to moderate	variable	strong
Cytoplasmic vacuolation	variable	variable	often prominent

Fig. 1.41   Summary of the morphological features of ALL of L1, L2 and L3 subtypes.

more difficult. The reproducibility of assignment into these two subtypes is improved if a scoring system such as that shown in Fig. 1.42[33] is used. Classification should be performed only on a well-spread and well-stained bone marrow film; classification based on peripheral blood morphology has been found to be less reliable[33].

Acute lymphoblastic leukaemia of L1 subtype

In L1 ALL[1], small cells, up to twice the diameter of a small lymphocyte, predominate. They have a high nucleo-cytoplasmic ratio. The nucleus is regular in shape with only occasional clefting or indentation, the chromatin pattern is fairly homogeneous, although smaller cells may show a greater degree of chromatin condensation, and the nucleoli, if visible at all, are small and inconspicuous. The scanty cytoplasm is slightly to moderately basophilic, rarely intensely basophilic, and in some cases shows a variable degree of vacuolation. In a minority of cases, small numbers of azurophilic granules are present.

Typical examples of L1 ALL are shown in Figs. 1.43 and 1.44. The L1 category includes the majority of cases of ALL; in childhood 70–80 percent of cases fall into this group. L1 ALL may be of B or T lineage.

Acute lymphoblastic leukaemia of L2 subtype

In L2 ALL[1] the blasts are larger and more heterogeneous. The nucleocytoplasmic ratio is variable from cell to cell but cytoplasm, which is variably basophilic, may be moderately abundant. The nucleus is irregular in shape, with clefting, folding and indentation being common, and with heterogeneity also of the chromatin pattern. Nucleoli are usually present and may be large. A variable degree of cytoplasmic vacuolation may be present, and in a minority of cases small numbers of azurophilic (but MPO-negative) granules are seen. Typical examples of L2 ALL are shown in Figs. 1.45–1.47. About one-quarter of cases of ALL fall into the L2 category. L2 ALL may be of B or T lineage.

Fig. 1.42 Scoring system for assigning ALL to L1 or L2 subtypes.

SCORING SYSTEM FOR ASSIGNING ALL TO L1 OR L2 SUBTYPES[33]

high nucleocytoplasmic ratio (cytoplasm less than 25 percent of the area of the cell) in at least 75 percent of cells	+1
low nucleocytoplasmic ratio (cytoplasm at least 20 percent of the area of the cell) in at least 25 percent of cells	−1
at least 75 percent of cells have no more than 1 small nucleolus	+1
at least 25 percent of cells have 1 or more prominent nucleoli	−1
nuclear outline irregular (reniform or grossly distorted by wide notches or pits) in at least 25 percent of cells	−1
large cells (diameter at least twice that of a small lymphocyte) comprise at least 50 percent	−1
A score of 0 to +2 indicates L1	
A score of −1 to −4 indicates L2	

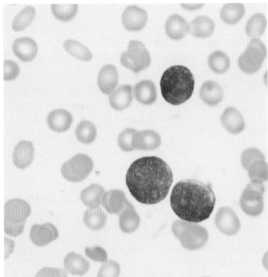

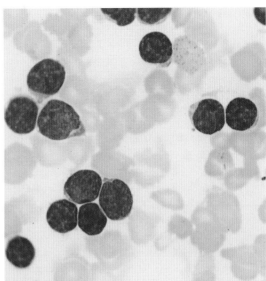

Fig. 1.43 PB film of a patient with L1 ALL. MGG × 960.

Fig. 1.44 BM film from a patient with L1 ALL. MGG × 960.

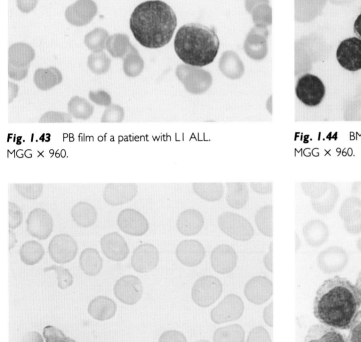

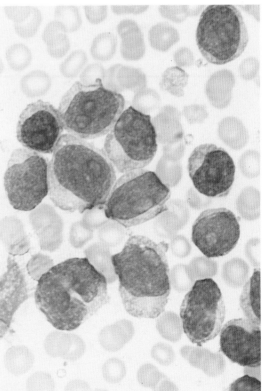

Fig. 1.45 BM film from a patient with L2 ALL showing large pleomorphic blasts; the cells were CD10 (common ALL antigen) positive. MGG × 960.

Fig. 1.46 BM film from a patient with L2 ALL showing medium to large pleomorphic blasts which were CD10 negative but positive for CD19, Ia and TdT. MGG × 960.

Acute lymphoblastic leukaemia of L3 subtype

In L3 ALL[1] the blast cells are large but homogeneous. The nucleocytoplasmic ratio is lower than in L1. The nucleus is regular in shape, varying from round to somewhat oval. The chromatin pattern is uniformly stippled or homogeneous, with one or more prominent, sometimes vesicular, nucleoli. In contrast to L1 and L2 ALL where mitotic figures are rarely seen, the mitotic index is high. The cytoplasm is strongly basophilic with variable but prominent vacuolation. Typical examples of L3 ALL are shown in Figs. 1.48–1.50. L3 ALL constitutes only 1–2 percent of ALL cases.

ALL of L3 subtype may be regarded as the leukaemic equivalent of Burkitt's lymphoma, since an aspirate performed on a lymph node or other tissue affected by this lymphoma shows cells which are morphologically the same as those of L3 ALL. 'Acute leukaemia with Burkitt's lymphoma cells' was first described in 1972[34], although the occurrence of bone marrow infiltration and a terminal leukaemic phase in endemic African Burkitt's lymphoma had been recognized prior to this.

The great majority of cases of L3 ALL have a mature B-cell phenotype, that is they have surface membrane immunoglobulin (SmIg). Rare cases have a common ALL phenotype, a pre-B phenotype (cytoplasmic immunoglobulin)[35] or even a T-cell[36] or hybrid T-B phenotype[37]. Cases have also been reported of acute leukaemia with L3 morphology with a lack of B or T markers, but with the characteristics of very early erythroid cells[38,39]; as these cases had the cytogenetic findings usually associated with L3 ALL/Burkitt's lymphoma (see page 71), the involvement of a primitive cell with the potential for both B-lymphoid and erythroid differentiation is suggested. Rarely, L3 morphology may be found in association with acute myelomonocytic leukaemia or undifferentiated carcinoma[40].

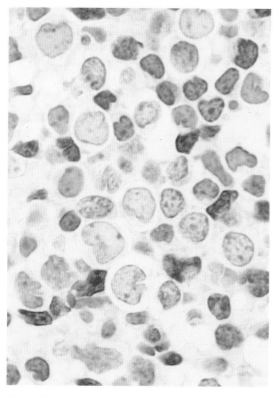

Fig. 1.47 Trephine biopsy of a patient with L2 ALL. Plastic embedded, H&E × 960.

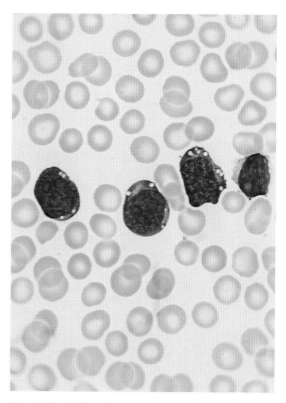

Fig. 1.48 PB film of a patient with L3 ALL with B-cell immunological phenotype. MGG × 960.

CYTOCHEMISTRY OF ALL

There is very little relationship between cytochemical reactions and the FAB categories, but somewhat more between cytochemical reactions and immunological categories of ALL.

Lymphoblasts show negative reactions with MPO and CAE stains. With SBB, very fine positive cytoplasmic granules may be present, but these are usually obscured by the counterstain so that for practical purposes SBB staining of blasts is negative[14]; these very fine granules probably represent mitochondria. Rare cases of apparent ALL have shown coarse granular positivity with SBB[14,41]. In ALL the neutrophils are MPO positive and show their normal strongly-positive staining with SBB, whereas in AML there may be a population of SBB-negative and MPO-negative neutrophils.

In B-lineage ALL, the PAS stain often shows a characteristic block positivity; this is seen also, though perhaps less often, in T-lineage ALL (Figs. 1.51 and 1.52). The blocks and coarse granules of positively staining material are present in cytoplasm which is completely PAS negative, whereas in the case of the block positivity which is seen much less often in cases of AML (mainly in monoblasts or erythroblasts), the PAS-positive blocks are in cells with a background diffuse or finely granular positivity (see Fig. 1.28b). L3 ALL is usually PAS negative[42].

In a recent study of 733 children with ALL[43], it was found that 28 percent of cases had more than 10 percent of vacuolated blasts. This finding correlated strongly with PAS positivity, a relatively low white cell count, and the presence of the common ALL antigen (CALLA). When cases had both vacuoles and PAS positivity, the chance of CALLA being positive was 98 percent. Although PAS staining is useful in the diagnosis of ALL, it is important to recognize that PAS block-positivity alone is not a sufficient basis for this diagnosis.

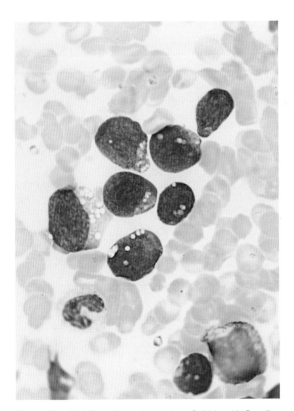

Fig. 1.49 BM film of a patient with L3 ALL with B-cell immunological phenotype. MGG × 960.

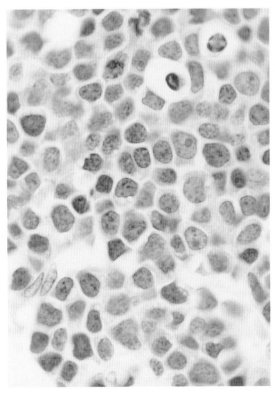

Fig. 1.50 Trephine biopsy from a patient with L3 ALL, B-cell phenotype; vacuolation of some of the blasts can be observed. Paraffin embedded, H&E × 960.

The presence of a strong, localized positivity for acid phosphatase is common in T-lineage ALL (Fig. 1.53), but rare in B-lineage ALL. This pattern should not, however, be regarded as pathognomonic for T-lineage ALL as a similar reaction is not uncommon in M6 AML, and may also be seen in M7 AML[17]. In a minority of cases of ALL the presence of azurophilic cytoplasmic granules on the Romanowsky stain can be related to the presence of lysosomal granules which also show punctate acid phosphatase activity[44]. This phenomenon correlates with B-lineage ALL (mainly cALL) and with L2 morphology. T lymphoblasts may also have localized coarse granular positivity for nonspecific esterase (NASDA, ANAE and ANBE), whereas B-lineage blasts either give negative reactions or have scattered fine granules. Neither pattern resembles the strong generalized positivity which is characteristic of cells of monocyte lineage.

In L3 ALL the vacuoles stain with Oil Red O, demonstrating that they contain lipid[42]. However Oil Red O-positive vacuoles may also be seen in L1 and L2 ALL, and were also noted in the case of metastatic carcinoma which simulated L3 ALL[40].

CLINICAL CORRELATES OF FAB CATEGORIES OF ACUTE LYMPHOBLASTIC LEUKAEMIA

ALL of L3 subtype is a distinct entity with a prognosis that is worse than that of other subtypes of ALL, although it is improving with modern treatment. Many cases cannot be distinguished clinically from other cases of ALL, but some show bone tumours, including very occasionally the jaw tumours that are characteristic of endemic African Burkitt's lymphoma[42]. L3 ALL together with Burkitt's lymphoma has recently been recognized as part of the spectrum of lymphoproliferative disorders associated with the acquired immunodeficiency syndrome (AIDS)[45].

L1 and L2 ALL clearly differ from L3 ALL, but the differences between the former two subtypes are less distinct. There is a difference in age distribution; L1 has its peak incidence in childhood and the incidence falls off rapidly with increasing age, while the incidence of L2 ALL does not vary much with age. The prognosis of L2 ALL is generally found to be worse than that of L1 ALL,

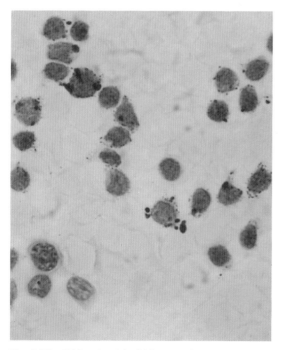

Fig. 1.51 PAS stain of the BM of a patient with common ALL showing block positivity. × 960.

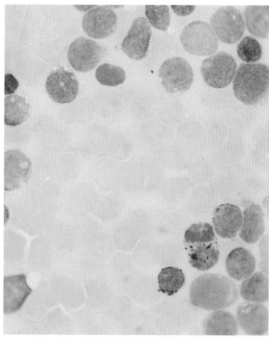

Fig. 1.52 PAS stain of the BM of a patient with T-ALL, L1 subtype, showing block positivity and showing positive granules on a clear background. × 960.

but in adults the difference is minor and lessens or disappears if the greater prognostic import of age is considered.

Patients with L2 morphology who relapse continue to have L2 morphology, but patients who initially have L1 morphology can relapse as L1 or L2[46]. Rarely L1 relapses as L3; in such cases cytogenetic study may show associated clonal evolution[47]. L3 ALL usually relapses as L3.

PROBLEMS WITH THE FAB CLASSIFICATION

A number of criticisms of the FAB classification have been made[5,6] which are summarized and discussed below.

Not all cases of acute leukaemia will be recognized if the requirement is accepted that blasts must constitute at least 30 percent of nucleated bone marrow cells or (in the case of M6 AML) of nonerythroid marrow cells.

Since leukaemia arises from transformation in a single cell, all cases of acute leukaemia necessarily pass from a stage when leukaemic cells are well below 1 percent of total bone marrow cells to a stage when leukaemic cells have largely replaced normal cells. The great majority of patients do not present to medical attention until the latter stage is reached but some, particularly those with pre-existing marrow dysfunction due to myelodysplasia, present with a lower proportion of blasts. The FAB classification is an attempt to standardize practice, but it is inevitable that any arbitrary cut-off point will misclassify some patients. Some cases which would have been categorized as M2 AML on the original FAB criteria[1], which required at least 50 percent of bone marrow cells to be blasts plus promyelocytes, do not have sufficient blasts to fit the revised criteria[4,8] for AML.

Diagnostic difficulty occurs mainly in patients with myelodysplasia, but occasionally in patients with *de novo* AML. Patients may either have a rapidly rising blast count but fewer than 30 percent blasts at the point when they present, or there may be maturation of leukaemic cells so that the blast percentage is low. The latter phenomenon is seen in M5b[5], M4[48] and M2 AML. For example, Dalton *et al.*[48] described two patients with acute myelomonocytic leukaemia associated with bone marrow eosinophilia and an abnormality of chromosome 16 (see page 76) who had only 21 and 28 percent, respectively, of bone marrow blasts, although circulating blast cell

counts were 42 and 73 $\times$ 10^9/l, respectively. Similar observations have been made for M2/t(8;21) AML. Recognition of specific haematological, morphological and cytogenetic features will often allow such cases to be recognized as AML, and they should be categorized as such. If there is any real diagnostic difficulty, the occurrence of progressive disease during a period of observation will permit the diagnosis to be made. In patients with features of myelodysplasia, consideration must be given to the rate of progression of the disease as well as to the blast percentage.

In M3 AML it is usually the case that blasts are less than 30 percent of bone marrow nucleated cells since the predominant cell is the abnormal hypergranular promyelocyte[1]. The distinctive morphology means that no practical problem occurs in making a diagnosis.

Not all cases of AML will be recognized as myeloid if the requirement for at least 3 percent of blasts to be positive for MPO or SBB is accepted.

As discussed on page 5, a wider definition of 'myeloid' is required to cover all classes of AML. It also seems desirable that cases of acute leukaemia in which the cells show minimal evidence of myeloid differentiation (see page 3) should be classified as myeloid not as lymphoblastic. However, when special tests are not available, adherence to the original FAB criteria[1] is justified since this will ensure that patients with lymphoblastic leukaemia in whom the chance of cure is significant are not misclassified as M0 and denied the most appropriate treatment.

Not all cases of acute myeloid leukaemia can be classified by the criteria of the FAB classification.

Some cases of acute leukaemia fit the FAB criteria for AML, but cannot be further classified since they do not exactly fit the criteria of any of the categories[6,27,49]. Unclassifiable cases are much more frequent among patients with secondary AML than among those with *de novo* AML[25,49,50,51]. In the Fourth International Workshop on Chromosomes in Leukaemia, the overall incidence of unclassifiable cases was about 2 percent, with 13 percent of cases of secondary leukaemia being unclassifiable, as opposed to less than 1 percent of *de novo* AML[50]. Unclassifiable cases have also been noted to be more common when AML occurs in a patient who has previously suffered from polycythaemia rubra vera[52] and in AML associated with the t(1;3) translocation[53].

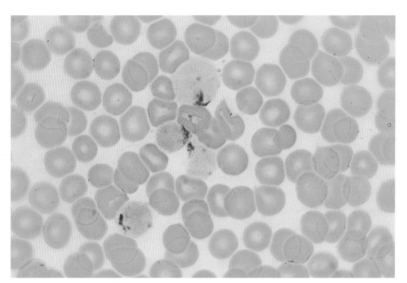

Fig. 1.53 Acid phosphatase stain of the PB of a patient with T-ALL (same patient as in Fig. 1.52) showing focal positivity. × 960.

The FAB categories are not reproducible.

There are some FAB categories, such as M3 and L3, which have such distinctive features that they yield a high concordance rate between observers. There are other categories which are less homogeneous and distinctive so that categorization is less reliable. Problems arise in distinguishing between L1 and L2, between M1 and M2, and between M2 and M4. Accuracy of categorization depends also on the experience and skill of the observer. In the Fourth International Workshop on Chromosomes in Leukaemia the overall rate of agreement between referring centre and final refereed category was 84 percent, but this varied between centres from 71 to 98 percent[50]. In other studies in AML, concordance rates have varied from 58 percent[54] to 87 percent[55]. In ALL, the problems with poor concordance between observers led the FAB group to introduce a scoring system to assign cases to L1 and L2 categories[33] (see Fig. 1.42).

In considering the often less than optimal concordance between observers attempting to apply the FAB criteria, one must bear in mind the level of concordance likely to be achieved if different observers assign cases to categories such as myeloblastic leukaemia, monoblastic leukaemia, myelomonocytic leukaemia and erythroleukaemia without the benefit of any definition or guidelines. The Eastern Cooperative Oncology Group compared their performance at such categorization before and after the introduction of the original FAB criteria and found an improvement from 48 to 61 percent[56].

The FAB classification is illogical.

It has been pointed out by Hayhoe[6] that it is illogical that different stages of maturation within the granulocyte lineage are assigned to different FAB categories (M1, M2), whereas different stages of maturation within the monocyte lineage are subsumed within one category (M5a and M5b), and no allowance is made for mature and immature variants of M4. This lack of logic does not create any practical problems.

The FAB classification is arbitrary and other dividing lines between classes would have been preferable.

In achieving the aim of standardization, not only between haematologists but also between countries, some clear-cut dividing lines between categories had to be drawn. Although the FAB group sought to recognize true entities, there is necessarily an element of arbitrariness in the choice of criteria. When it is found that a specific cytogenetic abnormality is associated with morphologically distinctive features and yet cases fall into more than one FAB category, it seems reasonable to conclude that such cases form a true entity and their division between two FAB categories is artificial and arbitrary; this is true, for example, for the cases with t(6;9) translocation associated with basophilia which may be classified as M2 or M4 (see page 78). The criteria for M6 have also been criticized[5,6], and it has been suggested that cases with between 30 and 50 percent of erythroid cells should be included in M6 when the erythroid lineage shows marked morphological abnormality[5]. The criteria for separating AML from myelodysplasia have likewise been criticized; this will be discussed in Chapter 2 (see page 58).

Despite problems which may be seen in current definitions of categories, it is desirable that changes in the classification should be kept to a minimum and confined to those that appear essential, or the comparability of series of cases reported at different times is lost.

The FAB classification does not allow for bilineage leukaemias.

It is now known that in a minority of acute leukaemias there are cells of both myeloid and lymphoid lineage (bilineage leukaemia), and in other cases there are cells which have features of both myeloid and lymphoid differentiation (biphenotypic leukaemia). Leukaemias of these types often cannot be suspected on the basis of morphology and cytochemistry alone. Their diagnosis requires relatively complex laboratory tests. The recognition of bilineage and biphenotypic leukaemias is clearly desirable when facilities are available since this diagnosis may be important for both prognosis and treatment[57]. When there are two morphologically distinct cell populations, a dual FAB classification can be used (for example M5b/L2).

The FAB classification excludes important information about cases which may be more biologically relevant than morphology and cytochemistry, for example cytogenetic and immunological characteristics, and evidence of multilineage involvement.

In the case of AML, some of the FAB categories are heterogeneous, partly by virtue of characteristics which are not considered in the FAB classification. For example, the M2 category brings together cases as diverse and prognostically different as *de novo* leukaemias arising in a granulocyte/monocyte-committed stem cell associated with the t(8;21) translocation (see page 72), and secondary leukaemias arising in a multipotent stem cell associated with abnormalities of chromosomes 5 and 7 and trilineage myelodysplasia. Factors of biological relevance, and often also of prognostic importance which are not included in the FAB categorization include the

degree of maturation of the leukaemic cells, whether the erythroid and megakaryocyte lineages are derived from the leukaemic clone, the presence and nature of cytogenetic abnormalities, immunological phenotype, and whether the leukaemia is secondary to radiotherapy/chemotherapy or arises *de novo*. It has been suggested that some of these features are of more relevance than the predominant cell type which is the basis of the FAB system[6].

Differentiation of leukaemic cells is indicated not only by the presence of maturing cells of the granulocyte and monocyte lineages, but also by the presence of granules or Auer rods in blast cells. Several studies have shown that the presence of Auer rods indicates a better prognosis[58,59,60]. The presence of granulocytic maturation as evidenced by Auer rods or Sudanophilia, or of monocytic differentiation as evidenced by nonspecific esterase activity, may be prognostically more important than the FAB category[6].

Whether or not the erythroid and megakaryocyte lineages are involved in the leukaemic process in cases classified as M1, M2, M4 and M5 appears to be prognostically important[6]. The poor prognosis of therapy-related AML and AML following myelodysplasia may relate at least in part to the characteristic trilineage involvement in these leukaemias. The presence of trilineage myelodysplasia (Figs. 1.54 and 1.55) in AML provides evidence for leukaemic transformation having occurred in a multipotent stem cell, and is associated with a poor prognosis[61]. Analysis of glucose-6-phosphate dehydrogenase (G6PD) alloenzyme patterns in erythrocytes and platelets also gives information as to whether these cells are derived from cells of the leukaemic clone, but this analysis is applicable to only a small minority of patients. PAS positivity of erythroblasts suggests that at least the erythroid lineage is part of the leukaemic clone and this has also been found to be prognostically important[60].

The presence and nature of cytogenetic abnormalities is undoubtedly of great importance (see Chapter 3), and studies of immunological markers are now starting to yield information of prognostic significance.

It is thus clear that there is indeed information of biological relevance which is not considered in the FAB classification. However, the perceived weakness of the classification, that it is based only on morphology and cytochemistry, is also its strength. As initially described[1], this classification could be applied by every haematologist in every laboratory, and with the exception of the recognition of the M7 category this remains true. Cytogenetic analysis is not yet available for all patients and in some

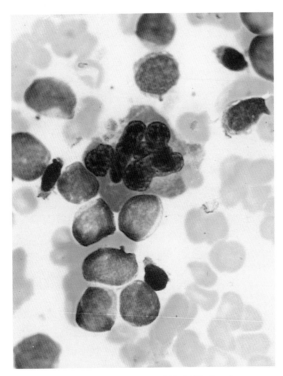

Fig. 1.54 BM of a patient with M1 AML showing a giant erythroid cell. MGG × 960.

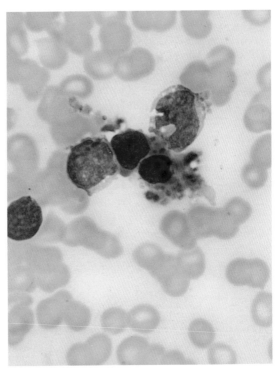

Fig. 1.55 BM of a patient with M4 AML showing two micromegakaryocytes (small round nucleus megakaryocytes). MGG × 960.

parts of the world it will remain unavailable in the foreseeable future. To a lesser extent this is also true of analysis of immunological markers of cell lineage. The introduction of the FAB classification has certainly led to improved communication between haematologists and it is likely, though not open to proof, that the standard of diagnosis has improved. The clearly defined categories have provided a framework for the presentation of information on cytogenetic abnormalities and have been useful in defining cytogenetic-clinicopathological correlations.

However, although morphology and cytochemistry remain the mainstay of haematological diagnosis, the major importance of information provided by more sophisticated techniques can hardly be underestimated. It is likely that further valuable advances in knowledge will follow from the characterization of cytogenetic abnormalities in acute leukaemia and from the search for oncogenes.

The study of immunological markers is also important in clarifying the nature of problem cases and in identifying unsuspected bilineage/biphenotypic leukaemia. It is clearly desirable that cases of acute leukaemia should be characterized as fully as possible. The FAB morphological classification can be easily integrated with immunological phenotype or with cytogenetic categories (see Chapter 3). It is much harder to integrate information on lineage involvement and cell differentiation without creating a large number of subcategories. Hayhoe has proposed an alternative classification[6] based on these two factors rather than on predominant cell type; this classification, which is summarized in Fig. 1.56, has not yet won general acceptance.

In ALL the role of immunological markers is more established than it is in AML, and clinical features, immunological phenotype and cytogenetic abnormalities are of more significance for prognosis and choice of treatment than is the FAB classification. An integrated classification based on FAB category, immunological phenotype and cytogenetic category can be used (see page 71).

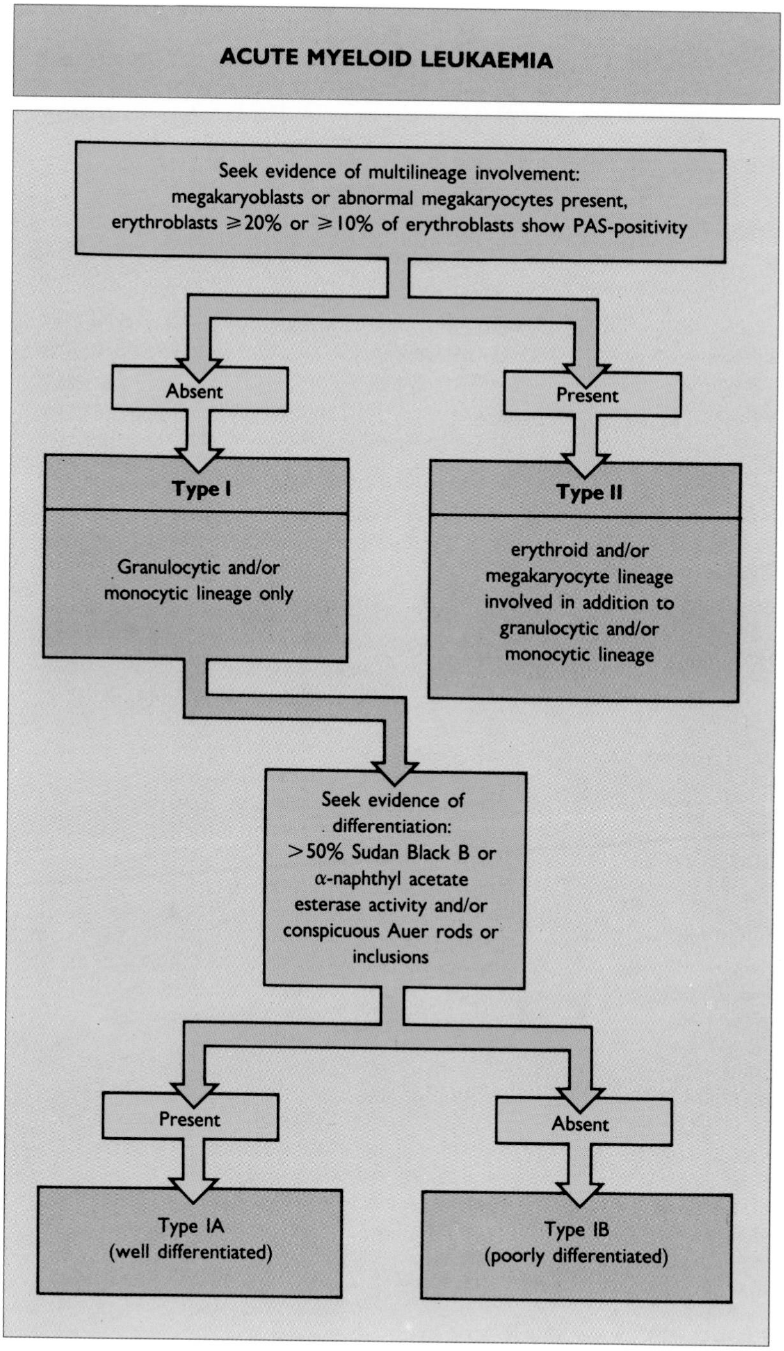

Fig. 1.56 A diagrammatic representation of an alternative classification of acute myeloid leukaemia proposed by Hayhoe[6].

ACUTE MYELOID LEUKAEMIA

Seek evidence of multilineage involvement: megakaryoblasts or abnormal megakaryocytes present, erythroblasts ≥20% or ≥10% of erythroblasts show PAS-positivity

Absent

Present

Type I

Granulocytic and/or monocytic lineage only

Type II

erythroid and/or megakaryocyte lineage involved in addition to granulocytic and/or monocytic lineage

Seek evidence of differentiation: >50% Sudan Black B or α-naphthyl acetate esterase activity and/or conspicuous Auer rods or inclusions

Present

Absent

Type IA (well differentiated)

Type IB (poorly differentiated)

REFERENCES

1. Bennett JM, Catovsky D, Daniel MT, Flandrin G, Galton DAG, Gralnick HR & Sultan C (1976) Proposals for the classification of the acute leukaemias (FAB cooperative group). *British Journal of Haematology*, **33**, 451–458.
2. Bennett JM, Catovsky D, Daniel MT, Flandrin G, Galton DAG, Gralnick HR & Sultan C (1980) A variant form of acute hypergranular promyelocytic leukaemia (M3). *British Journal of Haematology*, **44**, 169–170.
3. Bennett JM, Catovsky D, Daniel M-T, Flandrin G, Galton DAG, Gralnick HR & Sultan C (1985) Criteria for the diagnosis of acute leukemia of megakaryocytic lineage (M7): a report of the French–American–British cooperative group. *Annals of Internal Medicine*, **103**, 460–462.
4. Bennett JM, Catovsky D, Daniel MT, Flandrin G, Galton DAG, Gralnick HR & Sultan C (1985) Proposed revised criteria for the classification of acute myeloid leukemia. *Annals of Internal Medicine*, **103**, 620–629.
5. Bloomfield CD & Brunning RD (1985) The revised French–American–British classification of acute myeloid leukemia: Is new better? *Annals of Internal Medicine*, **103**, 614–616.
6. Hayhoe FGJ (1988) Classification of acute leukaemias. *Blood Reviews*, **2**, 186–193.
7. Galton DAG & Dacie JV (1975) Classification of the acute leukaemias. *Blood Cells*, **1**, 17–24.
8. Bennett JM, Catovsky D, Daniel MT, Flandrin G, Galton DAG, Gralnick HR & Sultan C (1982) Proposals for the classification of the myelodysplastic syndromes. *British Journal of Haematology*, **51**, 189–199.
9. Bain BJ (1989) *Blood cells: a practical guide*. Gower Medical Publishing, London.
10. Lee EJ, Pollak A, Leavitt RD, Testa JA & Schiffer CA (1987) Minimally differentiated acute nonlymphocytic leukemia; a distinct entity. *Blood*, **70**, 1400–1406.
11. Matutes E, de Oliveira MP, Foroni L, Morilla R & Catovsky D (1988) The role of ultrastructural cytochemistry and monoclonal antibodies in clarifying the nature of undifferentiated cells in acute leukaemia. *British Journal of Haematology*, **69**, 205–211.
12. Parreira A, de Oliviera MSP, Matutes E, Foroni L, Morilla R & Catovsky D (1988) Terminal deoxynucleotidyl transferase positive acute myeloid leukaemia: an association with immature myeloblastic leukaemia. *British Journal of Haematology*, **69**, 219– 224.
13. Imamura N & Kuramoto A (1988) Acute unclassifiable leukaemia in adults, demonstrating myeloid antigens and myeloperoxidase proteins. *British Journal of Haematology*, **69**, 427–428.
14. Hayhoe FGJ & Quaglino D (1988) *Haematological Cytochemistry, second edition*. Churchill Living stone, Edinburgh.
15. Yam LT, Li CY & Crosby WH (1971) Cytochemical identification of monocytes and granulocytes. *American Journal of Clinical Pathology*, **55**, 283–290.
16. Parkin JL, McKenna RW & Brunning RD (1982) Philadelphia-positive blastic leukaemia; ultrastructural and ultracytochemical evidence of basophil and mast cell differentiation. *British Journal of Haematology*, **52**, 663–677.
17. Polli N, O'Brien M, Tavares de Castro J, Matutes E, San Miguel JF & Catovsky D (1985) Characterization of blast cells in chronic granulocytic leukaemia in transformation, acute myelofibrosis and undifferentiated leukaemia. *British Journal of Haematology*, **59**, 277– 296.
18. Breton-Gorius J, Van Haeke D, Pryzwansky KB, Guichard J, Tabilio A, Vainchenker W & Carmel R (1984) Simultaneous detection of membrane markers with monoclonal antibodies and peroxidatic activities in leukaemia: ultrastructural analysis using a new method of fixation preserving the platelet peroxidase. *British Journal of Haematology*, **58**, 447–458.
19. Wick MR, Li C-Y & Pierre RV (1982) Acute nonlymphocytic leukemia with basophilic differentiation. *Blood*, **60**, 38–45.
20. Cawley JC & Hayhoe FGJ (1973) *The ultrastructure of haemic cells*. WB Saunders Company Ltd, London.
21. Matsuo T, Jain NC & Bennett JM (1988) Nonspecific esterase of acute promyelocytic leukemia. *American Journal of Hematology*, **29**, 148–151.
22. Testa JR, Golomb HM, Rowley JD, Vardiman JW & Sweet DL (1978) Hypergranular promyelocytic leukemia (APL): cytogenetic and ultrastructural specificity. *Blood*, **52**, 272–280.
23. Golomb HM, Rowley JD, Vardiman JW, Testa JR & Butler A (1980) "Microgranular" acute promyelocytic leukemia: a distinct clinical, ultrastructural and cytogenetic entity. *Blood*, **55**, 253–259.
24. McKenna RW, Parkin J, Bloomfield CD, Sundberg RD & Brunning RD (1982) Acute promyelocytic leukaemia: a study of 39 cases with identification of a hyperbasophilic microgranular variant. *British Journal of Haematology*, **50**, 201–214.
25. Berger R, Bernheim A, Daniel M-T, Valensi F & Flandrin G (1981) Karyotype and cell phenotypes in primary acute leukemias. *Blood Cells*, **7**, 287–292.
26. Scott CS, Patel D, Drexler HG, Master PS, Limbert HJ & Roberts BE (1989) Immunophenotypic and enzymatic studies do not support the concept of mixed monocytic–granulocytic differentiation in acute promyelocytic leukaemia (M3): a study of 44 cases. *British Journal of Haematology*, **71**, 505–509.
27. O'Brien M, Catovsky D & Costello C (1980) Ultrastructural cytochemistry of leukaemic cells. Characterization of the early small granules of monoblasts. *British Journal of Haematology*, **45**, 201–208.
28. Villeval JL, Cramer F, Lemoine A, Henri A, Bettaieb A, Bernaudin F, Beuzard Y, Berger R, Flandrin G, Breton-Gorius J & Vainchenker W (1986) Phenotype of early erythroblastic leukemias. *Blood*, **68**, 1167–1174.
29. Bain BJ, Catovsky D, O'Brien M, Spiers ASD & Richards HGH (1977) Megakaryoblastic transformation of chronic granulocytic leukaemia. *Journal of Clinical Pathology*, **30**, 235–242.
30. Breton-Gorius J, Reyes F, Vernant JP, Tulliez M & Dreyfus B (1978) The blast crisis of chronic granulocytic leukaemia: megakaryoblastic nature of cells revealed by the presence of platelet peroxidase – a cytochemical study. *British Journal of Haematology*, **39**, 295–303.
31. Bain BJ, Catovsky D, O'Brien M, Prentice HG, Lawlor E, Kumaran TO, McCann SR, Matutes E & Galton DAG (1981) Megakaryoblastic leukaemia presenting as acute myelofibrosis. A study of four cases with the platelet-peroxidase reaction. *Blood*, **58**, 206–213.
32. Fourth International Workshop on Chromosomes in Leukemia, 1982 (1984) Clinical significance of chromosome abnormalities in acute nonlymphoblastic leukemia. *Cancer Genetics and Cytogenetics*, **11**, 332–350.
33. Bennett JM, Catovsky D, Daniel MT, Flandrin G, Galton DAG, Gralnick HR & Sultan C (1981) The morphological classification of acute lymphoblastic leukaemia: concordance among observers and clinical correlations. *British Journal of Haematology*, **47**, 553–561.

34. Stevens DA, O'Conor GT, Levine PH & Rosen RB (1972) Acute leukemia with "Burkitt's lymphoma cells" and Burkitt's lymphoma. Simultaneous onset in American siblings; description of a new entity. *Annals of Internal Medicine*, **76**, 967–973.

35. Ganick DJ & Finlay JL (1980) Acute lymphoblastic leukemia with Burkitt cell morphology and cytoplasmic immunoglobulin. *Blood*, **56**, 311–314.

36. Koziner B, Mertelsmann R, Andreeff M, Arlin Z, Hansen H, de Harven E, McKenzie S, Gee T, Good R & Clarkson B (1980) Heterogeneity of cell lineages in L3 leukemias. *Blood*, **53**, 694–698.

37. Berman M, Minowada J, Loew JM, Ramsey MM, Ebie N & Knospe WH (1985) Burkitt cell acute lymphoblastic leukemia with partial expression of T-cell markers and subclonal chromosome abnormalities in a man with acquired immunodeficiency syndrome. *Cancer Genetics and Cytogenetics*, **16**, 341–347.

38. Ekblom M, Elonen E, Vuopio P, Heinonen K, Knuutila S, Gahmberg CG & Andersson LC (1982) Acute erythroleukaemia with L3 morphology and the 14q+ chromosome. *Scandinavian Journal of Haematology*, **29**, 75–82.

39. Knuutila S, Elonem E, Heinonen K, Borgström GH, Lakkala-Paranko T, Perkkiö M, Franssila K, Teerenhovi L, Ekblom M, von-Willebrand E, Jansson S-E, Almqvist A & de la Chapelle A (1984) Chromosome abnormalities in 16 Finnish patients with Burkitt's lymphoma or L3 acute lymphoblastic leukemia. *Cancer Genetics and Cytogenetics*, **13**, 139–151.

40. Castella A. Davey FR, Kurec AS & Nelson DA (1982) The presence of Burkitt-like cells in non-Burkitt's neoplasms. *Cancer*, **50**, 1764–1770.

41. Tricot G, Broeckaert-Van Orshoven A, Van Hoof A & Verwilghen RL (1982) Sudan Black B positivity in acute lymphoblastic leukaemia. *British Journal of Haematology*, **51**, 615–621.

42. Flandrin G, Brouet JC, Daniel MT & Preud'homme JL (1975) Acute leukemia with Burkitt's tumor cells: a study of six cases with special reference to lymphocyte surface markers. *Blood*, **45**, 183–188.

43. Lilleyman JS, Hann IM, Stevens RF, Richards SM & Eden OB (1988) Blast vacuoles in childhood lymphoblastic leukaemia. *British Journal of Haematology*, **70**, 183–186.

44. Darbyshire PJ & Lilleyman JS (1987) Granular acute lymphoblastic leukaemia of childhood: a morphological phenomenon. *Journal of Clinical Pathology*, **40**, 251–253.

45. Bernheim A & Berger R (1988) Cytogenetic studies of Burkitt lymphoma-leukemia in patients with acquired immune deficiency syndrome. *Cancer Genetics and Cytogenetics*, **32**, 67–74.

46. Lilleyman JS, Britton JA & Laycock BJ (1981) Morphological metamorphosis in relapsing lymphoblastic leukaemia. *Journal of Clinical Pathology*, **34**, 60–62.

47. Abromowitch M, Williams DL, Melvin SL & Stass S (1984) Evidence for clonal evolution in pre-B leukaemia. *British Journal of Haematology*, **56**, 409–416.

48. Dalton WT, Ahearn MJ, Cork O, Trujillo JM, Keating MJ, McCredie KB, Freireich EJ, Stass SA (1987) Acute myelomonocytic leukemia associated with abnormalities of chromosome 16; a light and electron microscopic study. *Hematologic Pathology*, **1**, 105–112.

49. Berger R, Bernheim A, Daniel M-T, Valensi F & Flandrin G (1981) Karyotype and cell phenotypes in acute leukemia following other diseases. *Blood Cells*, **7**, 293–299.

50. Fourth International Workshop on Chromosomes in Leukemia, 1982 (1984) Correlation between morphology and karyotype. *Cancer Genetics and Cytogenetics*, **11**, 275–281.

51. Bennett JM, Moloney WC, Greene MH & Boice JD (1987) Acute myeloid leukemia and other myelopathic disorders following treatment with alkylating agents. *Hematologic Pathology*, **1**, 99–104.

52. Berger R, Bernheim A, Flandrin G, Dresch C & Najean Y (1984) Cytogenetic studies on acute nonlymphocytic leukemias following polycythemia vera. *Cancer Genetics and Cytogenetics*, **11**, 441–451.

53. Bloomfield CD, Garson OM, Volin L, Knuutila S, de la Chapelle A (1985) t(1;3) (p36;q21) in acute nonlymphocytic leukemia: a new cytogenetic-clinicopathologic association. *Blood*, **66**, 1409–1413.

54. Head DR, Cerezo L, Savage RA, Craven CM, Bickers JN, Hartsock R, Hosty TA, Saiki JH, Wilson HE, Morrison FS, Coltman CA, Hutton JJ (1985) Institutional performance in application of the FAB classification of acute leukemia. The Southwest Oncology Group experience. *Cancer*, **55**, 1979–1986.

55. Dick FR, Armitage JO & Burns CP (1982) Diagnostic concurrence in the subclassification of adult acute leukemia using French–American–British criteria. *Cancer*, **49**, 916–920.

56. Bennett JM & Begg CB (1981) Eastern Cooperative Oncology Group study of the cytochemistry of adult acute myeloid leukemia by correlation of subtypes with response and survival. *Cancer Research*, **41**, 4833–4837.

57. Cross AH, Goorha RM, Nuss R, Behm FG, Murphy SB, Kalwinsky DK, Raimondi S, Kitchingman GR & Mirro J (1988) Acute myeloid leukemia with T-lymphoid markers. *Blood*, **72**, 579–587.

58. Mertelsmann R, Thaler HT, To L, Gee TS, McKenzie S, Schauer P, Friedman A, Arlin Z, Cirrincione C & Clarkson B (1980) Morphological classification, response to therapy and survival in 263 adult patients with acute nonlymphoblastic leukemia. *Blood*, **56**, 773–781.

59. Zittoun R, Cadiou M, Bayle C, Suciu S, Solbu G & Hayat M (1984) Prognostic value of cytologic parameters in acute myelogenous leukemia. *Cancer*, **53**, 1526–1532.

60. Swirsky DM, de Bastos M, Parish SE, Rees JKH & Hayhoe FGJ (1986) Features affecting outcome during remission induction of acute myeloid leukaemia in 619 adult patients. *British Journal of Haematology*, **64**, 435–453.

61. Brito-Babapulle F, Catovsky D & Galton DAG (1987) Clinical and laboratory features of de novo acute myeloid leukaemia with trilineage myelodysplasia. *British Journal of Haematology*, **66**, 445–450.

chapter two

THE MYELODYSPLASTIC

SYNDROMES

THE NATURE OF THE MYELODYSPLASTIC SYNDROMES AND THEIR DIAGNOSIS

In the initial FAB classification of the acute leukaemias a group of conditions designated the dysmyelopoietic syndromes were recognized and divided broadly into chronic myelomonocytic leukaemia (CMML) and refractory anaemia with excess of blasts (RAEB)[1]. The latter condition included cases which would previously have been classified as 'preleukaemia', 'smouldering leukaemia', 'subacute leukaemia' or 'atypical leukaemia'. The dysmyelopoietic syndromes, renamed the myelodysplastic syndromes (MDS), were further described and classified in 1982[2], with the criteria for distinguishing between acute myeloid leukaemia (AML) and MDS being further refined in 1985[3]. The incidence of MDS is about 6-times that of AML. It has been estimated at 0.75/1000/year in those over 60[4].

The MDS are a closely related group of acquired bone marrow disorders characterized by ineffective and dysplastic haemopoiesis. These conditions are intrinsic to the bone marrow and progressive. They are consequent on the proliferation of an abnormal clone of cells which replaces normal haemopoietic cells. The MDS may either be apparently primary or may evolve in the course of other bone marrow diseases, or be secondary to previous exposure to cytotoxic chemotherapy, irradiation or other environmental toxins. The defect may be principally manifest in one lineage (the granulocytic/monocytic lineage, the erythroid lineage or, less often, the megakaryocyte lineage), but commonly dysplasia is bilineal or trilineal. There is usually a discrepancy between a cellular or hypercellular bone marrow and peripheral blood cytopenia, although in up to 10 percent of cases the bone marrow is hypocellular. Although cytopenia is most characteristic, some patients exhibit neutrophil leucocytosis, monocytosis, thrombocytosis or, rarely, eosinophilia or basophilia.

Dysplastic haemopoiesis is not confined to the MDS, being seen, for example, during the administration of certain drugs and in megaloblastic anaemia. The diagnosis of MDS requires the recognition of features consistent with this diagnosis and the elimination of alternative causes. Haematological abnormalities which may occur are shown in Fig. 2.1. The usefulness of such features in diagnosis varies. Some abnormalities, such as an acquired Pelger–Huët anomaly (Fig. 2.2) or micromegakaryocytes (defined here as megakaryocytes less than 20 μm in diameter) (Fig. 2.3), are highly characteristic and almost pathognomonic of MDS; one or other of these abnormalities occurs in a high percentage of patients[5]. Agranular neutrophils (Fig. 2.4) are also highly specific but are present in a smaller proportion of patients. Other abnormalities such as macrocytosis, monocytosis or neutropenia are less specific, and require that alternative diagnoses be eliminated. In some patients the features at presentation may not be sufficient to make a firm diagnosis, but as disease progression occurs the diagnosis becomes certain.

The diagnosis of a myelodysplastic syndrome may be aided by ferrokinetic studies to demonstrate ineffective erythropoiesis, studies with monoclonal antibodies to demonstrate aberrant antigen expression, cytochemistry (see page 54), bone marrow histology (see page 54), bone marrow culture (see page 55) and cytogenetic analysis to demonstrate an acquired clonal abnormality (see page 80).

HAEMATOLOGICAL ABNORMALITIES WHICH MAY OCCUR IN THE MYELODYSPLASTIC SYNDROMES

Erythropoiesis

Peripheral blood
anaemia
   normocytic normochromic (common)
   macrocytic (common)
   microcytic (uncommon)
dimorphic blood film
anisocytosis, poikilocytosis
   (which may include ovalocytes, tear drop
   poikilocytes, schistocytes, stomatocytes)
circulating nucleated red blood cells
   which may show dyserythropoietic or
   megaloblastic features or may be ring sideroblasts
   with defective haemoglobinization
Pappenheimer bodies
basophilic stippling

Bone marrow
hyperplasia (common)
hypoplasia (uncommon)
megaloblastic erythropoiesis
macronormoblastic erythropoiesis
sideroblastic erythropoiesis
dysplastic erythropoiesis
   with features such as binuclearity, multi-nuclearity,
   nuclear lobulation, nuclear fragmentation,
   increased Howell–Jolly bodies, inter-nuclear
   bridges, gaps in nuclear membrane, increased
   pyknosis, gigantism

Granulopoiesis

Peripheral blood
neutropenia (common)
neutrophilia (uncommon)
acquired Pelger–Huët anomaly
neutrophils with hypersegmented nuclei, increased
   nuclear projections, ring nuclei or nuclei of
   bizarre shape; increased chromatin clumping in
   neutrophils or precursors
agranular and hypogranular neutrophils
hypergranular neutrophils
persistence of cytoplasmic basophilia in mature cells
Döhle bodies
monocytosis
abnormal monocytes
promonocytes
blast cells, with or without Auer rods
eosinophilia (uncommon)
hypogranular eosinophils and eosinophils with ring-
   shaped nuclei or non-lobulated nuclei
basophilia (uncommon)

Bone marrow
granulocytic hyperplasia
granulocytic hypoplasia
increased blast cells, with or without Auer rods
hypogranular or hypergranular promyelocytes
hypogranular myelocytes
increase of monocytes and promonocytes
lack of mature neutrophils
morphologically abnormal neutrophils
increased eosinophils (uncommon)
increased basophils (uncommon)

Thrombopoiesis

Peripheral blood
thrombocytopenia (common)
thrombocytosis (uncommon)
giant platelets
agranular platelets
platelets with giant granules
micromegakaryocytes*

Bone marrow
reduction of megakaryocytes
increase of megakaryocytes
mononuclear or binuclear micromegakaryocytes,*
   larger megakaryocytes with nonlobed nuclei,†
   multinucleated megakaryocytes, megakaryocytes
   with botryoid nuclei

*The term micromegakaryocyte has been used in various senses. It was used first to describe the megakaryocytes of CGL but the megakaryocytes which are most characteristic of MDS are <20 μm in diameter[5], much smaller than the characteristic forms of CGL. MDS megakaryocytes are typically small with a small round nucleus; they could perhaps be termed SRN megakaryocytes. †Abnormal megakaryocytes characteristic of the 5q− syndrome are >30 μm and have a large round nucleus; they could be termed LRN megakaryocytes; the term "large mononuclear megakaryocyte" should be avoided since normal megakaryocytes are both large and mononuclear.

Fig. 2.1 Haematological abnormalities which may occur in the myelodysplastic syndromes.

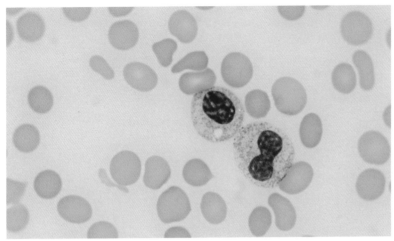

Fig. 2.2 PB film of a patient with refractory anaemia secondary to cytotoxic chemotherapy showing the acquired Pelger–Hüet anomaly; also apparent are anisocytosis, poikilocytosis and severe thrombocytopenia. The BM showed trilineage myelodysplasia. MGG × 960.

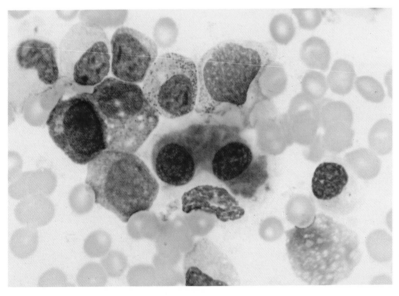

Fig. 2.3 Micromegakaryocytes in the BM of a patient with refractory anaemia; there was also granulocytic hyperplasia, hypogranularity of the neutrophil series and severe erythroid hypoplasia. MGG × 960.

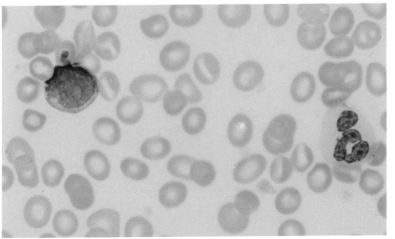

Fig. 2.4 Agranular neutrophil in the PB of a patient with refractory anaemia with excess of blasts. One myeloblast is present, some red cells are stomatocytic and platelet numbers are markedly reduced. MGG × 960.

The MDS need to be distinguished from the myelo-proliferative disorders, amongst which are included polycythaemia rubra vera, essential thrombocythaemia, idiopathic myelofibrosis and chronic myeloid leukaemia. In the myeloproliferative disorders, haemopoiesis is generally effective and excessive, with erythrocytosis, thrombocytosis, neutrophilia and basophilia being common whereas in myelodysplasia, haemopoiesis is generally ineffective with increased cell death in the marrow leading to various cytopenias. There is, however, some overlap between the two groups of diseases. CMML shares many features with other members of the myelo-dysplastic group, but it resembles other chronic myeloid leukaemias in that production of monocytes and neutro-phils is effective, and hepatomegaly and splenomegaly are common. The childhood syndrome associated with monosomy 7[6] is usually regarded as a myeloproliferative disorder but has some features of myelodysplasia. Some patients with refractory anaemia and some with sidero-blastic anaemia have effective production of platelets so that thrombocytosis rather than thrombocytopenia is seen. Although most patients with the 5q− syndrome[7,8] (see page 48) are anaemic and are regarded as having myelodysplasia, a minority initially present as essential thrombocythaemia without anaemia. Both the myelo-proliferative and the myelodysplastic disorders may terminate in acute leukaemia. Myelodysplasia may super-vene in patients with myeloproliferative disorders and the likelihood of acute leukaemia is then greatly increased. Myelodysplastic features such as hypogranular and hypolobulated granulocytes often develop during the course of myelofibrosis. Sideroblastic erythropoiesis, the acquired Pelger–Huët anomaly and diploid megakaryo-cytes may appear during transformation of CGL and may herald blast crisis. Similarly, in some patients with polycythaemia rubra vera a myelodysplastic phase precedes the development of acute leukaemia.

It is likely that the great majority if not all cases of MDS arise through a genetic alteration in a multipotent stem cell. This is suggested by studies of G6PD allo-enzymes[9], by cytogenetic analysis[10], and by investigation of *ras* oncogene mutations and active and inactive al-leles of X chromosome genes[11]. Lineages which appear morphologically normal may be part of the abnormal clone, and in some cases the T lymphocytes[10] or both T and B lymphocytes[9,11] are also clonal; lymphocytopenia is common in MDS. The myelodysplastic clone is un-stable, and with the passage of time clonal evolution occurs. This is often associated with the acquisition of new karyotypic abnormalities and shows itself in pro-gressive marrow failure, an increase in the number of blast cells or the development of overt acute leukaemia, which is usually myeloid but occasionally lymphoblastic.

The FAB classification of the MDS is based on morpho-logy of the blood and bone marrow, supplemented by a cytochemical stain for iron. It is summarized in Fig. 2.5. In applying the classification (Fig. 2.6), the most impor-tant features are the numbers of blast cells and the presence of Auer rods. When the peripheral blood blast cells reach 5 percent or the bone marrow blast cells exceed 20 percent or Auer rods are present, the case is classified as refractory anaemia with excess of blasts in transformation (RAEB-t) irrespective of other features. In classifying the remaining cases the number of mono-cytes is assessed. If the peripheral blood monocyte count exceeds $1 \times 10^9/l$ the case is classified as CMML regard-less of other features such as the sideroblast percentage. Following allocation to the RAEB-t and CMML cate-gories, remaining cases are classified on the basis of the numbers of blasts and ring sideroblasts. If the peripheral blood blasts exceed 1 percent or the bone marrow blasts reach 5 percent, the case is categorized as RAEB. If blasts have not reached these levels but bone marrow sidero-blasts exceed 15 percent of erythroblasts, the case is classified as refractory anaemia with ring sideroblasts (RARS). If there is neither an excess of blasts nor more than 15 percent ring sideroblasts, the case is refractory anaemia (RA). It will be noted that the monocyte count may exceed $1 \times 10^9/l$ in both CMML and RAEB-t, and the sideroblast count may exceed 15 percent in all categories except RA. The FAB classification of MDS is often applied incorrectly and it is sometimes stated that there is overlap between the categories. If the criteria are applied correctly, as summarized here, there is no ambiguity or overlap in the classification.

Refractory anaemia

About 30–40 percent of cases of MDS are classed as RA (Figs. 2.2 and 2.3). Commonly, the patient presents with symptoms of anaemia or the diagnosis is an incidental one. A minority of patients have hepatomegaly or splenomegaly.

The patient is anaemic and there is an absolute reticulocytopenia. Red cells are commonly macrocytic but sometimes normocytic. Some anisocytosis and poi-kilocytosis may be present, together with some basophilic stippling. In macrocytic cases the degree of anisocytosis is less than that which is seen in megaloblastic anaemia, and oval macrocytes are not usual.

THE FAB CLASSIFICATION OF THE MYELODYSPLASTIC SYNDROMES		
Category	**peripheral blood**	**bone marrow**
Refractory anaemia (RA) or refractory cytopenia*	anaemia,* blasts $\leqslant$1% monocytes $\leqslant$1 $\times$ 10^9/l AND	blasts <5%, ring sideroblasts $\leqslant$15% of erythroblasts
Refractory anaemia with ring sideroblasts (RARS)	anaemia, blasts $\leqslant$1% monocytes $\leqslant$1 $\times$ 10^9/l AND	blasts <5%, ring sideroblasts >15% of erythroblasts
Refractory anaemia with excess of blasts (RAEB)	anaemia monocytes $\leqslant$1 $\times$ 10^9/l blasts >1% OR	blasts $\geqslant$5%
	blasts <5% AND	blasts $\leqslant$20%
Chronic myelomonocytic leukaemia (CMML)	monocytes >1 $\times$ 10^9/l, granulocytes often increased, blasts <5%	blasts up to 20%, promonocytes often increased
Refractory anaemia with excess of blasts in transformation (RAEB-t)	blasts $\geqslant$5% OR Auer rods in blasts in blood or marrow OR	blasts >20% BUT blasts <30%
Or in the case of refractory cytopenia either neutropenia or thrombocytopenia*		

Fig. 2.5 The FAB classification of the myelodysplastic syndromes[2,3].

In some cases morphological and quantitative abnormalities are confined to the red cell series, but other patients are neutropenic or thrombocytopenic, or show pseudo-Pelger–Huët (Fig. 2.2) or hypogranular neutrophils, or large or agranular platelets. Thrombocytosis is occasionally seen, particularly in patients with the 5q– chromosomal anomaly. Occasional blasts may be present, but they do not exceed 1 percent and monocytes do not exceed 1 $\times$ 10^9/l.

In the majority of patients the bone marrow is hypercellular; in a minority is is normocellular or hypocellular. Erythropoiesis is dysplastic and either normoblastic, macronormoblastic or megaloblastic. Rarely there is a virtually complete red cell aplasia (Fig. 2.3). Ring sideroblasts may be present but do not exceed 15 percent. Iron stores are often increased. Some cases show dysplastic granulopoiesis and thrombopoiesis (Fig. 2.3). Bone marrow blasts are less than 5 percent.

A significant proportion of patients with RA have deletion of the long arm of chromosome 5 (5q–) as the sole cytogenetic abnormality, and have characteristics which have been designated the 5q– syndrome[7]. There is a female preponderance, macrocytic anaemia, hypolobulated megakaryocytes and a relatively good prognosis. The abnormal megakaryocytes have nonlobed or bilobed nuclei but are mainly more than 30–40 µm in diameter (Fig. 2.7)[8]; they thus differ from the mononuclear and binuclear micromegakaryocytes (see Fig. 2.2) associated with other forms of MDS which are no larger than other haemopoietic cells. Some patients with the 5q– syndrome fall into the RARS or RAEB categories.

OTHER REFRACTORY CYTOPENIA

Some patients with MDS are cytopenic but not anaemic and do not fit into any of the other categories of MDS. They are grouped with the refractory anaemias and are designated refractory cytopenia. Both refractory neutropenia and refractory thrombocytopenia occur. Refractory

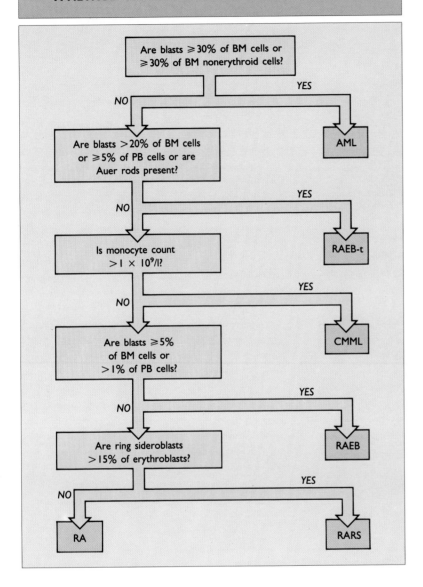

Fig. 2.6 A method of applying the FAB classification[2,3].

A METHOD OF APPLYING THE FAB CLASSIFICATION[2,3]

thrombocytopenia may constitute 3–4 percent of patients with MDS. The peripheral blood may show large or hypogranular platelets while the bone marrow shows an increase of megakaryoblasts and micromegakaryocytes. In some cases platelet life span is somewhat reduced but thrombocytopenia is mainly a consequence of ineffective production of platelets.

REFRACTORY MACROCYTOSIS

Some patients with MDS are macrocytic but not anaemic. If they do not have an excess of monocytes, ring sideroblasts or blasts it seems reasonable that they should be designated refractory macrocytosis and should be grouped with RA.

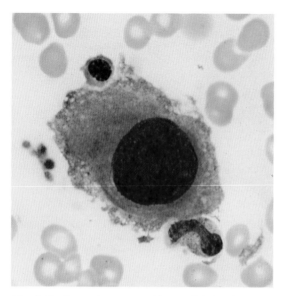

Fig. 2.7 A megakaryocyte with a nonlobulated nucleus in the BM of a patient with the 5q– syndrome. MGG × 960.

Refractory anaemia with ring sideroblasts

RARS, also designated primary acquired sideroblastic anaemia, constitutes 15–25 percent of MDS. Usually either the patient presents with symptoms of anaemia or the diagnosis is made incidentally. The serum iron is usually high, with increased transferrin saturation and a high serum ferritin concentration.

The patient is anaemic with the red cells commonly being macrocytic but sometimes normocytic or microcytic. The mean cell volume (MCV) is usually normal or high, but occasionally reduced. The blood film (Fig. 2.8) is often dimorphic with a predominant population of normochromic macrocytes and a minor population of hypochromic microcytes. Basophilic stippling may be present. A careful search usually reveals the presence of Pappenheimer bodies (Fig. 2.8), particularly within hypochromic cells. A small number of circulating nucleated red blood cells can often be found, and it may be noted that they show defective haemoglobinization and sometimes basophilic cytoplasmic granules adjacent to the nucleus. An iron stain will confirm the nature of Pappenheimer bodies and thus positively identify siderocytes and ring sideroblasts. Neutropenia, thrombocytopenia or dysplastic changes in neutrophils or platelets may be present, but often these lineages are morpho-

logically and quantitatively normal. A minority of patients with sideroblastic anaemia have thrombocytosis. Occasionally blast cells are present in the peripheral blood but they are not more than 1 percent. The monocyte count does not exceed $1 \times 10^9/l$.

The bone marrow (Fig. 2.9) is generally hypercellular with erythroid hyperplasia and dyserythropoiesis. Erythropoiesis may be normoblastic, macronormoblastic or megaloblastic, with an appreciable percentage of erythroblasts showing either ragged, scanty cytoplasm or more ample cytoplasm which is defectively haemoglobinized and contains granules (Fig. 2.9). On an iron stain, ring sideroblasts are readily identified (Fig. 2.10) and constitute more than 15 percent of erythroblasts. There is also an increase of other abnormal sideroblasts in which the iron-containing granules are increased in size and number but are not disposed in a ring. In primary acquired sideroblastic anaemia, siderotic granules are often present in early erythroid cells from basophilic erythroblasts onwards, whereas in hereditary or secondary sideroblastic anaemia the changes are confined to late erythroblasts. Ultrastructural examination shows that in ring sideroblasts the iron is deposited in mitochondria, whereas in other abnormal sideroblasts, and in the sideroblasts of normal bone marrow, iron is in cytoplasmic micelles. Iron stores are commonly increased. This may be a feature of other categories of MDS in advance of any transfusion therapy but it is commonest in sideroblastic anaemia. If a patient with sideroblastic anaemia develops coincidental severe iron deficiency, the percentage of ring sideroblasts falls in most but not all cases, and rarely ring sideroblasts totally disappear only to reappear when iron stores are replenished. Patients with sideroblastic anaemia may have dysgranulopoiesis or dysthrombopoiesis, but often these cell lines are morphologically normal. Bone marrow blasts are less than 5 percent.

Refractory anaemia with excess of blasts

RAEB constitutes 15–25 percent of MDS. Patients usually present with symptoms of anaemia or with infection or bruising.

Patients with RAEB may show the red-cell features of either RA or RARS. Neutropenia, thrombocytopenia, and dysplastic changes in neutrophils and platelets are more common in RAEB than in the latter two conditions. Peripheral blood blast cells are usually present (Fig. 2.4) but are less than 5 percent. The monocyte count is not greater than $1 \times 10^9/l$.

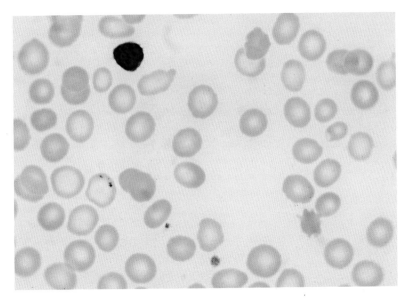

Fig. 2.8 PB film of a patient with idiopathic acquired sideroblastic anaemia (RARS). The blood film is dimorphic and one red cell contains Pappenheimer bodies. Poikilocytes including an acanthocyte are present. Pappenheimer bodies are basophilic iron-containing granules which can be distinguished from basophilic stippling by being larger, more peripherally situated and less frequent within a cell. MGG × 960.

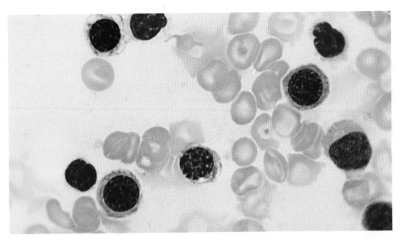

Fig. 2.9 BM film in a patient with idiopathic acquired sideroblastic anaemia (RARS) showing erythroid hyperplasia but only slight dyserythropoiesis. One erythroblast shows defective haemoglobinization and has basophilic granules within its cytoplasm. MGG × 960.

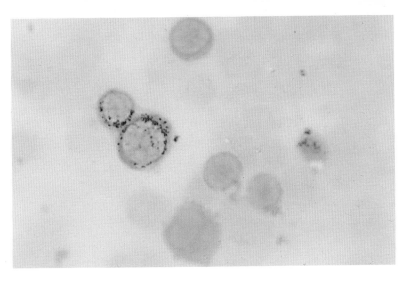

Fig. 2.10 BM film of a patient with sideroblastic anaemia (same patient as Fig. 2.9) stained by Perls' reaction for iron. Two ring sideroblasts are present. × 960.

The bone marrow blasts are usually increased to at least 5 percent but do not exceed 20 percent; in those cases without 5 percent of bone marrow blasts the peripheral blood blasts must be greater than 1 percent for the criteria of RAEB to be met. Blasts are often small with scanty cytoplasm and are undifferentiated on an MGG stain. Bilineage or trilineage myelodysplasia is more common in RAEB than in RA or RARS. Ring sideroblasts may be present and may exceed 15 percent of erythroblasts.

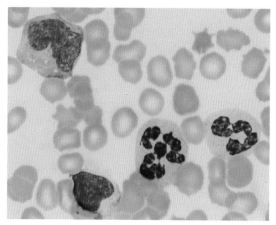

Fig. 2.11 PB film of a patient with CMML showing a monocyte, a lymphocyte and two neutrophils, one of which has a nucleus of abnormal shape. The red cells are poikilocytic and platelet numbers are reduced. × 960.

The FAB designation 'refractory anaemia with excess of blasts' is preferred to 'refractory anaemia with excess of myeloblasts' since the blasts present are not invariably myeloblasts.

Chronic myelomonocytic leukaemia

CMML constitutes about 15 percent of MDS. Patients usually present with symptoms of anaemia, with the clinical picture of leukaemia, or with both. Anaemia is less common than in RA or RARS, whereas hepatomegaly and splenomegaly are much more common than in other types of myelodysplasia. A minority of patients have pleural, pericardial or peritoneal effusions, synovitis, lymphadenopathy or skin infiltration[4,12]. Rarely gum hypertrophy occurs[4]. Serum lysozyme is usually elevated, and urinary lysozyme sometimes. Rare cases of renal failure may be related to elevated urinary lysozyme[13]. Associated immunological dysfunction is common. Immunoglobulin concentrations are elevated in about one-third of patients, and 5–10 percent have a monoclonal protein. Autoantibodies are present in about one-half of patients; these may include cold agglutinins. The direct antiglobulin test is positive in about 10 percent of cases. (Immunological abnormalities may occur in other categories of MDS but they appear to be commonest in CMML.)

The peripheral blood (Fig. 2.11) shows a monocyte count of greater than 1×10^9/l. Monocytes are some-

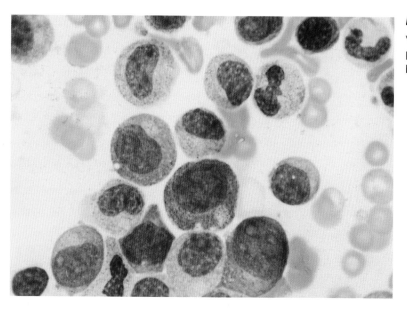

Fig. 2.12 BM film of a patient with CMML, showing predominantly granulocytic hyperplasia. × 960.

times morphologically abnormal with hypersegmented or bizarre-shaped nuclei, or with features of immaturity such as increased basophilia and some cytoplasmic granules. Some promonocytes may be present but monoblasts are rarely seen. The neutrophil count is usually also elevated but this is not essential for the diagnosis. Neutrophils sometimes show dysplastic features. Anaemia may be present and is usually normocytic and normochromic. Macrocytosis may also occur and in patients with sideroblastic erythropoiesis, hypochromic microcytes and a dimorphic blood film are present. Occasional patients with a positive direct antiglobulin test have haemolysis with spherocytes on the blood film. Those with an increase of immunoglobulins, either polyclonal or monoclonal, usually have increased rouleaux formation and an elevated erythrocyte sedimentation rate. The platelet count may be normal or low and dysplastic features may be present. Peripheral blood blasts are less than 5 percent.

The bone marrow (Fig. 2.12) is hypercellular. Promonocytes are prominent with relatively few mature monocytes. In some cases there is marked granulocytic hyperplasia with monocyte precursors being inconspicuous. Blasts vary from low levels to 20 percent. Ring sideroblasts may be present and may exceed 15 percent of the erythroblasts. Dysplastic features may be observed in all lineages but in some patients with CMML dysplasia in erythroid and megakaryocyte lineages is minimal.

CMML requires separation not only from other MDS but also from other chronic myeloid leukaemias. There is no difficulty in distinguishing it from Ph-positive chronic granulocytic leukaemia since this condition shows few dysplastic features prior to transformation and has a very characteristic peripheral blood film (see page 106). The distinction from atypical Ph-negative CML is more difficult, but this latter condition has a much worse prognosis than CMML and the distinction appears valid. Atypical CML may also show some dysplastic features. The most useful distinguishing feature is the presence of appreciable numbers of myelocytes, and usually promyelocytes and blasts, in CML. A cut-off point of 15 percent of immature granulocytes has been suggested to make the distinction, but in the great majority of cases there are fewer than 5 percent[14]. Eosinophilia and basophilia are sometimes present in atypical CML but are very unusual in CMML, with the exception of secondary cases which sometimes show basophilia.

Refractory anaemia with excess of blasts in transformation

Patients with RAEB-t (Fig. 2.13) usually present with symptoms of anaemia and with infection and haemorrhage. Hepatomegaly and splenomegaly may be present.

The peripheral blood may show 5 percent or more blasts, or blasts containing Auer rods. Any of the other features described in the other MDS may be present, with anaemia, neutropenia, thrombocytopenia and dysplastic neutrophils and platelets being usual. Some patients

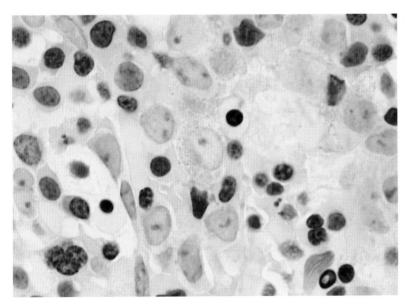

Fig. 2.13 Trephine biopsy from a patient with RAEB-t showing erythroblasts, some of which are dyserythropoietic, blasts and promyelocytes. H&E, × 960.

have monocytosis. The bone marrow blasts are usually above 20 percent but less than 30 percent. To meet the criteria for RAEB-t, either peripheral blood or bone marrow blasts must be increased or Auer rods must be present (see Fig. 2.5). Trilineage myelodysplasia is usual in RAEB-t.

CYTOCHEMICAL REACTIONS IN THE MYELODYSPLASTIC SYNDROMES

The only cytochemical reaction essential in the diagnosis and classification of the MDS is a Perls' stain for iron which is necessary for assessing the presence and number of ring sideroblasts. Other cytochemical reactions may provide evidence of dysplastic maturation and can thus be useful both in confirming the diagnosis and in assessing the number of lineages involved. In CMML, staining for nonspecific esterase activity may be necessary to identify the monocytic component in the bone marrow[1]. As in AML, Auer rods may occasionally be demonstrated only by cytochemical stains.

Cytochemical stains for MPO, naphthol AS-D chloro-acetate esterase (CAE) and SBB may show mature neutrophils with negative reactions[15], and similarly mature monocytes may be deficient in nonspecific esterase activity. Particularly in CMML, individual cells may show reactivity for both CAE and nonspecific esterase, activities normally characteristic of granulocytic and monocytic lineages respectively. The NAP score is reduced in one-third to one-half of patients, and is elevated in a minority.

When patients with MDS have an increase of bone marrow blasts the cells show the cytochemical reactions expected of myeloblasts, monoblasts or megakaryoblasts. Relatively undifferentiated myeloblasts are the form most commonly present so that positive reactions for SBB, MPO and CAE may be weak and confined to a minority of cells. In some cases the blasts do not give positive reactions with any cytochemical markers of myeloid cells. Such cases are generally M0 blasts, but in a minority of cases the cells appear to be lymphoblasts.

Erythroblasts may be PAS positive, with the positive reaction being confined to proerythroblasts or being present in early, intermediate and late erythroblasts[16]. Although PAS positivity is seen in some reactive conditions, its presence in patients with MDS or leukaemia is likely to indicate that the lineage is part of the abnormal clone. Erythroblasts may also show aberrant strong para-nuclear positivity for acid phosphatase and nonspecific

esterase; such reactions are not confined to MDS and AML but may be seen in megaloblastic anaemia[15]. In MDS both the percentage of haemoglobin F and the cells containing haemoglobin F may be increased. A cyto-chemical stain such as the Kleihauer reaction will identify the increased percentage of haemoglobin F-containing cells. Such an increase is not confined to MDS.

BONE MARROW BIOPSY

Bone marrow aspiration and trephine biopsy are com-plementary investigations. Biopsy often gives extra information which is not provided by an aspirate[17,18,19]. Cellularity can be more reliably assessed and increased reticulin is apparent. Abnormal distribution of cells is often detectable. Erythroid islands may be absent or may show an excess of proerythroblasts or have all precursors at the same stage of development[17]. Granulocytic pre-cursors may be clustered centrally rather than showing their normal paratrabecular distribution. This pheno-menon has been designated 'Abnormal Localization of Immature Precursors' (ALIP)[17]. This can be diagnostically important if it is detected in RA since its presence con-firms MDS rather than a secondary anaemia. Abnormal megakaryocytes (mononuclear, binuclear and multi-nucleated forms) are readily assessed on a biopsy. Dysgranulopoiesis and dyserythropoiesis, including the presence of ring sideroblasts, may be detectable but they are more readily apparent in a bone marrow film. If, as sometimes occurs, all the iron has been removed from a biopsy specimen by a decalcification process, ring sidero-blasts will of course be undetectable. Biopsies may show nonspecific abnormalities such as prominent mast cells, lymphoid follicles and plasma cell aggregates.

The experience of different groups differs as to whether FAB subtypes of MDS constitute recognizable histological entities. Tricot et al.[17] could not recognize entities which corresponded to the FAB categories. Delacrétaz et al.[19], however, reached concordant diag-noses in 24 of 28 cases examined independently. Both groups found ALIP in more than half the biopsies, but Tricot et al.[18] found it in all subtypes of MDS (though preferentially in RAEB and RAEB-t), whereas Delacrétaz et al.[19] found ALIP to be very uncommon in those cases which did not have an excess of blasts in the aspirate.

Biopsy is particularly useful in assessing cases with a normocellular or hypocellular bone marrow and cases with increased reticulin in which a poor aspirate, which is unlikely to be representative, is obtained. It is particularly likely to be useful, therefore, in secondary MDS in which both reduced cellularity and increased reticulin are much more common than in primary MDS. Biopsy is helpful in distinguishing hypocellular MDS, which may have increased reticulin and foci of blasts, from aplastic anaemia which does not show these features.

BONE MARROW CULTURE

There is some correlation between the FAB categories and the results of bone marrow culture. A normal growth pattern of CFU-GM is most often seen in RA and RARS, whereas an abnormal pattern is usual in CMML, RAEB and RAEB-t. The abnormal pattern may be either reduced colonies, increased colonies and/or clusters (the commonest pattern in CMML) or reduced colonies and increased clusters (in some, but not all, studies predictive of transformation to acute leukaemia). Growth of BFU-E, CFU-E and CFU-Meg is often reduced or absent but shows no correlation with FAB subtype.

EVOLUTION OF THE MYELODYSPLASTIC SYNDROMES

Patients with MDS may die of marrow failure as a direct consequence of the MDS or may die following transformation to acute leukaemia. The likelihood of either outcome and the rapidity with which it occurs varies in the different FAB categories, so that both the percentage of patients developing acute leukaemia and the prognosis as reflected in the median survival differ significantly between FAB categories (Figs. 2.14 and 2.15). Myelo-dysplastic syndromes may also evolve into other myelo-dysplastic syndromes. Change is usually into a worse prognostic category and very rarely into a more favourable category. Thus RA and RARS may evolve into either CMML or RAEB, both of which may in turn evolve into RAEB-t. Variation in the number of monocytes can alter the classification, mainly between CMML and RAEB; rarely ring sideroblasts disappear so that RARS converts to RA. When acute leukaemia supervenes it may develop within a brief period, or a stepwise evolution over many weeks or months may be apparent. The acute leukaemia which occurs in MDS is almost always AML, but rare cases of ALL and of bilineage/biphenotypic leukaemia have been reported; this occurrence is consistent with the evidence suggesting that, in at least some cases, the cell which gives rise to the MDS clone is a pluripotent stem cell capable of both myeloid and lymphoid differentiation. Since MDS is predominantly a disease of the elderly, a significant proportion of patients with MDS die of other diseases. The likelihood of this outcome is of course greatest in those in the best prognostic categories, RA and RARS. Occasional patients with MDS, particularly with RA and RARS, die of iron overload.

MEDIAN SURVIVAL IN MONTHS IN THE FAB CATEGORIES OF MYELODYSPLASIA						
Number of cases	RA	RARS	CMML	RAEB	RAEB-t	Reference
101	20	14	4	13	2.5	28
141	32	76	22	10.5	5	21
109	64	71	8	7	5	29
237	50	>60	>60	9	6	30
107	23	31	9.4	8	4	31

This figure includes only data from series containing more than 100 patients and in which the FAB criteria have been applied with minor or no modifications.

Fig. 2.14 Median survival in months in the FAB categories of MDS.

THE PERCENTAGE OF PATIENTS TRANSFORMING TO ACUTE LEUKAEMIA IN THE FAB CATEGORIES OF MYELODYSPLASIA							
Number of cases	Length of follow-up	RA	RARS	CMML	RAEB	RAEB-t	Reference
141	4 months– 16 years	11	5	13	28	55	21
109	4–9 years	15	0	32	27	50	29
256	5 years	26	16	17	66	60	30
101	"long term"	16	7	0	38	47	28

This figure contains data only from series containing more than 100 patients and in which the FAB criteria have been applied with minor or no modifications.

Fig. 2.15 The percentage of patients transforming to acute leukaemia in the FAB categories of MDS.

PROGNOSIS OF THE MYELODYSPLASTIC SYNDROMES

A number of factors can be correlated with prognosis in the MDS (Fig. 2.16). The FAB classification divides patients into two broad prognostic groups, RA plus RARS and RAEB plus RAEB-t. There is no consistent or statistically significant difference between median survivals in RA and RARS, although leukaemic transformation is less common in RARS[20] (Figs. 2.14 and 2.15). The prognosis of RAEB-t is somewhat worse than that of RAEB and in large series the difference in survival becomes significant[20]. The prognosis of CMML has been variable between different series of patients (Fig. 2.14).

There is considerable heterogeneity within FAB categories and efforts have been made to use other criteria to give a clearer idea of prognosis in the individual patient. The Bournemouth Score[21,12] (Fig. 2.17) is recommended since it is easy to apply, is based on data readily available in all patients, and has been validated in several independent studies. (The utility of the modification introduced to indicate prognosis in CMML[12] was not, however, confirmed in one study[22].) The scoring system recently described by a Spanish cooperative group[20] may also prove useful. It was validated in a second set of patients and is simple to apply, requiring only age, platelet count and percentage of bone marrow blasts. The scoring system of Varela et al.[23] is much more complex to apply and does not offer any clear advantages over the Bournemouth or Spanish scores.

CRITICISMS WHICH HAVE BEEN MADE OF THE FAB CLASSIFICATION OF THE MYELODYSPLASTIC SYNDROMES

Some cases of myelodysplasia are omitted from the FAB classification.

This is true of patients with refractory macrocytosis consequent on myelodysplasia who are not anaemic and do not have monocytosis or an excess of ring sideroblasts which would allow them to be assigned to other categories[24]. It seems most appropriate that such patients should be designated 'refractory macrocytosis' and grouped with RA. It is likely that their prognosis is at least as good as that of cases of RA. Similarly, patients with sideroblastic erythropoiesis consequent on myelodysplasia are not always anaemic[25]; such cases can reasonably be grouped with sideroblastic anaemia. Patients with myelodysplasia who are not anaemic but have neutropenia or thrombocytopenia are not excluded from the FAB classification since refractory cytopenia is included in the RA group[2].

Some cases may be unclassifiable.

It has been stated that some cases of myelodysplasia cannot be classified using the FAB criteria. This has been reported to be common in secondary myelodysplasia[26] but has also been observed in primary myelodysplasia. The problem arises because of a reluctance to assign

FACTORS WHICH HAVE BEEN REPORTED TO BE OF PROGNOSTIC SIGNIFICANCE IN THE MYELODYSPLASTIC SYNDROMES

	factors indicating good prognosis	factors indicating poor prognosis
clinical features	younger female de novo MDS	older male secondary MDS splenomegaly (in CMML)
FAB category	RA or RARS	RAEB or RAEB-t
peripheral blood features		anaemia, neutropenia, thrombocytopenia, presence of blast cells, neutrophilia (in CMML), monocytosis (in CMML)
bone marrow aspirate		increased blast cells, dysgranulopoiesis, dysmegakaryopoiesis, reduced megakaryocytes
bone marrow trephine biopsy		abnormal localization of immature precursors (ALIP)
ferrokinetics	near normal iron utilization at 14 days	low iron utilization at 14 days, increased ineffective erythropoiesis
karyotype	normal, both normal and abnormal metaphases, 5q−, +8 or 20q− as sole abnormality	abnormalities of chromosome 7 or both 5 and 7, all metaphases abnormal, complex karyotype
bone marrow culture	normal numbers of CFU-GM colonies and clusters	reduced CFU-GM colonies or increased colonies and/or clusters
cell kinetics		low labelling index
biochemistry		elevated LDH

Fig. 2.16 Factors which have been reported to be of prognostic significance in the MDS.

patients with severe trilineage myelodysplasia to the RA or RARS categories, particularly in view of the FAB group's statement that in RA 'the granulocytic and megakaryocytic series almost always appear normal'[2]. However, the FAB group also pointed out that in RA and RARS they occasionally found morphological abnormalities in the granulocytic and megakaryocytic series identical with those present in other subtypes of MDS[2]. This is particularly likely to be true in secondary MDS. Although prominent trilineage dysplasia is likely to indicate a worse prognosis, such patients can nevertheless be assigned to the RA or RARS categories.

Other reports of unclassifiable patients relate to a belief that categories overlap and that there is therefore a problem in assigning patients to either RAEB or CMML or to either RARS or CMML. As explained on page 47 such overlap does not occur if the FAB classification is correctly applied.

If adequate diagnostic material is available and if the small numbers of nonanaemic, noncytopenic patients with dysplastic or sideroblastic erythropoiesis are included in the RA and RARS categories as suggested above, then all patients with MDS should be classifiable by FAB criteria.

THE MODIFIED BOURNEMOUTH SCORE – A SCORING SYSTEM FOR ASSESSING PROGNOSIS IN MYELODYSPLASIA[12,21]	
feature	score
haemoglobin concentration ≤ 10 g/dl	+ 1
platelet count ≤ 100 × 10⁹/l	+ 1
neutrophil count ≤ 2.5 × 10⁹/l	+ 1
neutrophil count* > 16 × 10⁹/l	+ 1
bone marrow blasts ≥ 5%	+ 1

score	prognosis	median survival**
0–1	good	62 months
2–3	intermediate	22 months
4	poor	8.5 months

* this criterion was added when Bournemouth score was modified[12]
** median survivals of 141 subjects analysed for unmodified Bournemouth score[21]

Fig. 2.17 The modified Bournemouth score – a scoring system for assessing prognosis in myelodysplasia[12,21]

A different problem occurs when it is not clear if a patient has myelodysplasia or a myeloproliferative disorder. This dilemma is not peculiar to the FAB classification but relates rather to the existence of patients whose features overlap these two groups of diseases (see page 47).

The FAB categories or the criteria for assigning patients to them are inappropriate.

It is possible to criticize the underlying concept of the FAB classification. Patients with MDS could be regarded as a single group of patients all with the same disease, with any division into separate categories or subtypes being arbitrary. There is some validity in this view since patients in one category will share characteristics with patients in another and many features which can be quantitated show a continuous range. Patients move from one category into another. Patients of the same subtype have diverse chromosomal abnormalities while the same chromosomal abnormality is found in different subtypes. Some histopathologists[17] have difficulty recognizing the FAB subtypes as entities and see many similarities between cases categorized differently. Despite these considerations there are major differences in the nature of the disease between different patients, and most haematologists feel a need to categorize in a manner

which relates both to haematological features and to prognosis. Being based only on morphology, the FAB classification can be used by all haematologists whereas classifications based, for example, on cytogenetics or immunological markers have a more limited availability. Although others have described or defined RAEB, CMML and primary sideroblastic anaemia, this is the only comprehensive classification. It has been widely accepted and seems unlikely to be replaced by any other in the near future.

In addition to criticizing the concept of the FAB classification, it is possible to question the criteria for assignment to subtypes.

RAEB-t.
Two criticisms which have been made in relation to the RAEB-t subtype are that it cannot be justified as a category since it comprises or contains patients whose prognosis is no worse than that of other patients with MDS and, conversely, that some patients with AML are mistakenly included in this group.

Soon after the publication of the FAB classification it was suggested that an increase of the blast count to between 20 and 30 percent was not significant and did not justify a separate category[27]. Subsequent publications have fairly consistently shown a worse median survival in

RAEB-t than in RAEB (see Fig. 2.14). Although this difference has not always reached statistical significance, few now doubt that RAEB-t has a worse prognosis than does RAEB. In fact the prognosis of RAEB-t is not much better than that of untreated AML. The assigning of cases to the RAEB-t category because of the presence of Auer rods has been criticized on two counts. Some have held that the presence of Auer rods is diagnostic of acute leukaemia and incompatible with MDS. Others have suggested the Auer rods do not alter the prognosis of patients with MDS and should therefore not be the sole basis for classifying patients as RAEB-t[32]. The poor prognostic significance of Auer rods has recently been supported by the observation that patients less than 20 years of age with numerous Auer rods, classified as RAEB-t, have a disease course very similar to that of AML and are more likely to respond well to chemotherapy than the majority of patients with MDS[33]. Other problems relating to deciding if a patient is correctly classified as RAEB-t or as AML have been discussed on page 37.

RARS.

It has been suggested that patients should be classified as having primary acquired sideroblastic anaemia, or RARS, when they have an excess of ring sideroblasts irrespective of other factors. Since the presence of blast cells is of greater prognostic significance than the presence of ring sideroblasts and since the presence or absence of sideroblasts does not alter the prognosis in patients with RAEB[34] or, in one study, MDS as a whole[20], it seems preferable to follow the FAB recommendations. Other cut-off points for a percentage of ring sideroblasts regarded as significant have been suggested, for example 20 percent rather than 15 percent of erythroblasts. Since there is a continuous range of sideroblast counts from nought to greater than 90 percent any cut-off point is necessarily somewhat arbitrary and there does not seem to be any good reason to choose another level. It should be mentioned that the FAB group actually suggested that ring sideroblasts should be counted as a percentage of all nucleated bone marrow cells rather than as a percentage of erythroblasts[3]; it seems likely that percentage of erythroblasts was intended and I have described the FAB classification on this basis.

CMML.

CMML appears to be a much more heterogeneous group than other categories of MDS. Reported median survival has varied greatly (see Fig. 2.14). It has been suggested that the number of monocytes should be ignored and cases of CMML should be reassigned to other categories[35]. Maintaining the category of CMML does, however, have the advantage of reminding haematologists that patients with MDS may have clinical and laboratory features more commonly associated with leukaemia, such as marked splenomegaly, infiltrative lesions and high white cell counts. It also serves to emphasize that the differential diagnosis of patients with 'leukaemia' and monocytosis includes MDS as well as atypical CML. Since the prognosis of atypical CML is generally considerably worse than that of CMML, the distinction is important.

Other levels of monocyte count have been suggested as the cut-off point for the diagnosis of CMML. There is a continuous range of monocyte counts in MDS, with higher counts being associated with a worse prognosis in some series. Any specific cut-off point is, therefore, to some extent arbitrary, but there is no clear advantage to choosing a different cut-off point, thereby destroying the comparability between different series of patients.

The FAB classification ignores other information of prognostic value.

The use of the FAB morphological classification does not preclude gathering and assessing other relevant information on the nature of the disease. This can be done within the framework of the FAB morphological classification and such proposals have been made by the Third MIC Cooperative Study Group[26]. It is also useful to assign a prognostic score such as the Bournemouth score[21,12] or the Spanish score[20] to each patient.

REFERENCES

1. Bennett JM, Catovsky D, Daniel MT, Flandrin G, Dalton DAG, Gralnick HR & Sultan C (1976) Proposals for the classification of the acute leukaemias (FAB cooperative group). *British Journal of Haematology*, **33**, 451–458.

2. Bennett JM, Catovsky D, Daniel MT, Flandrin G, Galton DAG, Gralnick HR & Sultan C (1982) Proposals for the classification of the myelodysplastic syndromes. *British Journal of Haematology*, **51**, 189–199.

3. Bennett JM, Catovsky D, Daniel MT, Flandrin G, Galton DAG, Gralnick HR & Sultan C (1985) Proposed revised criteria for the classification of acute myeloid leukemia. *Annals of Internal Medicine*, **103**, 626–629.

4. Hamblin TJ & Oscier DG (1987) The myelodysplastic syndromes – a practical guide. *Hematological Oncology*, **5**, 19–34.

5. Kuriyama K, Tomonaga M, Matsuo T, Ginnai I & Ichimaru M (1986) Diagnostic significance of detecting pseudo-Pelger–Huët anomalies and micromegakaryocytes in myelodysplastic syndrome. *British Journal of Haematology*, **63**, 665–669.

6. Evans JPM, Czepulkowski B, Gibbons B, Swansbury GJ & Chessels JM (1988) Childhood monosomy 7 revisited. *British Journal of Haematology*, **69**, 41–45.

7. van den Berghe H, Vermaelen K, Mecucci C, Barbieri D & Tricot G (1985) The 5q- anomaly. *Cancer Genetics and Cytogenetics*, **17**, 189–255.

8. Thiede T, Engquist L & Billstrom R (1988) Application of megakaryocyte morphology in diagnosing 5q- syndrome. *European Journal of Haematology*, **41**, 434–437.

9. Prchal JT, Throckmorton DW, Carroll AJ, Fuson EW, Gams RA & Prchal JF (1978) A common progenitor for human myeloid and lymphoid cells. *Nature*, **274**, 590–591.

10. Rashkind WH, Tirumali N, Jacobson R, Singer J & Fialkow PJ (1984) Evidence for a multistep pathogenesis of a myelodysplastic syndrome. *Blood*, **63**, 1318–1323.

11. Janssen JWG, Buschle M, Layton M, Drexler HG, Lyons J, van den Berghe H, Heimpel H, Kubanek B, Kleihauer E, Mufti GJ & Bartram CR (1989) Clonal analysis of myelodysplastic syndrome: evidence of multipotent stem cell origin. *Blood*, **73**, 248–254.

12. Worsley A, Oscier DG, Stevens J, Darlow S, Figes A, Mufti G & Hamblin TJ (1988) Prognostic factors of chronic myelomonocytic leukaemia. *British Journal of Haematology*, **68**, 17–21.

13. Solal-Celigny P, Desaint B, Herrera A, Chastang C, Amar M, Vroclans M, Brousse N, Mancilla F, Renoux M, Bernard J-F & Boivin P (1983) Chronic myelomonocytic leukemia according to the FAB classification analysis of 35 cases. *Blood*, **63**, 634–638.

14. Krsnik I, Srivastava PC & Galton DAG (1990), *Blut*, (in press).

15. Schmalzl F, Konwalinka G, Michlmayr G, Abbrederis K & Braunsteiner H (1978) Detection of cytochemical and morphological abnormalities in 'Preleukemia'. *Acta Haematologica*, **59**, 1–18.

16. Hayhoe FGJ & Quaglino D (1988) *Haematological Cytochemistry, Second Edition*, Churchill Livingstone, Edinburgh.

17. Tricot G, de Wolf Peeters C, Hendrickx B & Verwilghen RL (1984) Bone marrow histology in myelodysplastic syndromes. *British Journal of Haematology*, **56**, 423–430.

18. Tricot G, Vleitinck R, Boogaerts MA, Hendrickx B, de Wolf Peeters C, van den Berghe H & Verwilghen RL (1985) Prognostic factors in the myelodysplastic syndrome: importance of initial data on peripheral blood counts, bone marrow cytology, trephine biopsy and chromosomal analysis. *British Journal of Haematology*, **60**, 19–32.

19. Delacrétaz F, Schmidt P-M, Piguet D, Bachman F & Costa J (1987) Histopathology of myelodysplastic syndromes: the FAB classification. *American Journal of Clinical Pathology*, **87**, 180–186.

20. Sanz GF, Sanz MA, Vallespi T, Cañizo MC, Torrabadella M, Garcia S, Irriguible D & San Miguel JF (1989) Two regression models and a scoring system for predicting survival and planning treatment in myelodysplastic syndromes: a multivariate analysis of prognostic factors in 370 patients. *Blood*, **74**, 395–408.

21. Mufti GJ, Stevens JR, Oscier DG, Hamblin TJ & Machin D (1985) Myelodysplastic syndromes; a scoring system with prognostic significance. *British Journal of Haematology*, **59**, 425–433.

22. del Cãnizo MC, Sanz G, San Miguel JF, Vallespi T, Irriguible D, Torrabadelle M & Sanz MA (1989) Chronic myelomonocytic leukemia – clinicobiological characteristics: a multivariate analysis in a series of 70 cases. *European Journal of Haematology*, **42**, 466–473.

23. Varela BL, Chuang C, Woll JE & Bennett JM (1985) Modifications in the classification of primary myelodysplastic syndromes; the addition of a scoring system. *Hematological Oncology*, **3**, 55–63.

24. May SJ, Smith SA, Jacobs A, Williams A & Bailey-Wood R (1985) The myelodysplastic syndromes; analysis of laboratory characteristics in relation to the FAB classification. *British Journal of Haematology*, **59**, 311–319.

25. Bowen DT & Jacobs A (1989) Primary acquired sideroblastic erythropoiesis in non-anaemic and minimally anaemic subjects. *Journal of Clinical Pathology*, **42**, 56–58.

26. Third MIC Cooperative Study Group (1988) Recommendations for a morphologic, immunologic and cytogenetic (MIC) working classification of the primary and therapy-related myelodysplastic disorders. *Cancer Genetics and Cytogenetics*, **32**, 1–10.

27. Seigneurin D (1983) Refractory anaemia with excess of blasts in transformation: is a new category necessary? *British Journal of Haematology*, **55**, 196–197.

28. Vallespi T, Torrabadella M, Julio A, Irriguible D, Jaen A, Acebedo G & Triginer J (1985) Myelodysplastic syndromes: a study of 101 cases according to the FAB classification. *British Journal of Haematology*, **61**, 83–92.

29. Foucar K, Langdon RM, Armitage JO, Olson DB & Carroll TJ (1985) Myelodysplastic syndromes. A clinical and pathological analysis of 109 cases. *Cancer*, **56**, 553–561.

30. Kerkhofs H, Hermans J, Haak HL & Leeksma CHW (1987) Utility of the FAB classification for myelodysplastic syndromes: investigation of prognostic factors in 237 cases. *British Journal of Haematology*, **65**, 73–81.

31. Garcia S, Sanz MA, Amigo V, Colomina P, Carrera MD, Lorenzo JI & Sanz GF (1988) Prognostic factors in chronic myelodysplastic syndromes: a multivariate analysis. *American Journal of Hematology*, **29**, 163–168.

32. Weisdorf DJ, Oken MM, Johnson GJ & Rydell RE (1981) Auer rod positive dysmyelopoietic syndrome. *American Journal of Hematology*, **68**, 397–402.

33. Scoazec J-Y, Imbert M, Crofts M, Jouault H, Juneja SK, Vernant J-O & Sultan C (1985) Myelodysplastic syndrome or acute myeloid leukaemia? A study of 28 cases presenting with borderline features. *Cancer*, **55**, 2390–2394.

34. Yoshida Y, Oguma S, Uchino H & Maekawa T (1987) Significance of ring sideroblasts in refractory anaemia with excess of blasts. *British Journal of Haematology*, **65**, 119–120.

35. Bennett JM, Cox C, Moloney WC, Rosenthal DS & Storniolo AM (1988) Chronic myelomonocytic leukemia (myelodysplasia with monocytosis). *XXII Congress of the International Society of Hematology, Milan*, **Abstract Sym-M-3-6.**

chapter three IMMUNOLOGICAL, CYTOGENETIC AND OTHER MARKERS

INTRODUCTION

Morphology and cytochemistry are fundamental to the diagnosis and classification of the acute leukaemias and MDS, but important and often essential information is also gained from immunophenotyping and cytogenetic analysis.

In AML, immunophenotyping is particularly important in the diagnosis of M0 and M7 AML and of AML of early erythroid phenotype. The immunophenotype can form the sole basis of a classification of AML[1] but more often it is used in conjunction with morphology. When used to supplement the FAB classification there is an improvement both in accuracy and in concordance between observers[2].

Much of the cytogenetic information can be interpreted only in the light of the morphology since the same apparent chromosomal abnormality may be found in both acute and chronic leukaemia or in both MDS and AML. However there are some cytogenetic abnormalities which identify a subtype of AML with such high specificity that the subtype may be defined more accurately by the karyotype than by the morphology. Phenotypic and cytogenetic information can be combined with the FAB subtype to describe individual cases more fully and to divide patients into distinct groups with differing prognosis. Proposals for such classifications have been made by the MIC groups[3,4].

In ALL both immunophenotype and the presence and nature of a cytogenetic abnormality are more important from the point of view of prognosis and treatment than the FAB subtype. Immunophenotype can form the sole basis of a classification or can be integrated with the FAB category and karyotypic information as proposed by the

MIC group[3]. Immunophenotyping is essential for the identification of bilineage or biphenotypic leukaemia (see page 68).

IMMUNOLOGICAL MARKERS AND FAB SUBTYPES OF ACUTE LEUKAEMIA

Cell surface structures of normal leucocytes and leukaemic cells can be studied by means of rosetting techniques, for example with sheep erythrocytes (ERFC, a marker of T lymphocytes) or mouse erythrocytes (MRFC, a marker of a subset of B cells). Surface and cytoplasmic antigens can also be recognized by antibodies. Initially such antibodies were available as polyclonal antisera raised by the immunization of an animal, particularly a rabbit, with normal or leukaemic cells. Subsequently, the development of techniques to immortalize antibody-producing cells by hybridizing them with mouse myeloma cells permitted the production of monoclonal antibodies (McAb), the specificity of which was stable and could be defined.

This hybridoma technology has led to the wide availability of antibodies suitable for typing leukaemic cells and also made possible standardization of techniques. The laboratory methods currently employed depend mainly on such McAb although some polyclonal antisera are still in use. Most antibodies are clustered into groups with the same or very similar specificity, each cluster being indicated by a CD or cluster of differentiation number. Several standard panels for the initial phenotyping of acute leukaemia have been proposed[3,5,6]. The more important McAb used in acute leukaemia classification are shown in Figs. 3.1, 3.2 and also 3.5.

MONOCLONAL ANTIBODIES (McAb) USEFUL IN THE DIAGNOSIS AND CLASSIFICATION OF ACUTE LEUKAEMIA – THOSE IDENTIFYING MAINLY EARLY PRECURSOR CELLS AND CELLS OF B LINEAGE

Cluster of differentiation	Representative McAb	Specificity within haemopoietic lineage
unclustered	OKIa, GRB1, HLA-Dr, FMC4	major histocompatibility complex Class II antigens, HLA-Dr (Ia): B lymphocytes and B-lymphocyte progenitors, activated T lymphocytes, a small minority of T-lineage ALL (mainly in adults), monocytes, myeloid precursors, most AML
unclustered	anti-TdT*	terminal deoxynucleotidyl transferase in nucleus: ALL, 10–20 percent of AML
CD34	My10, 3C5	B-lineage lymphoblasts, early T-cell precursors[7], myeloid progenitors, myeloblasts
CD19	B4, Leu 12	B lymphocytes and B-lymphocyte precursors, B-lineage ALL
CD22	To15, Leu 14, RFB-4	B-lineage: as a surface antigen in B lymphocytes, as a cytoplasmic antigen in B-lymphocyte precursors, as a surface antigen in about 14 percent of B-lineage ALL and as a cytoplasmic antigen in about 98 percent[5]
CD24	BA-1	B lymphocytes and precursors, B-lineage ALL, granulocytes
CD20	B1, OKB7, Leu 16	B lymphocytes, some B-lymphocyte precursors, some B-lineage ALL
CD10	J5, OKB-CALLA, BA-3, VILA1	common ALL antigen (CALLA): a subset of B-cell progenitors, about 90 percent of B-lineage ALL, some T-lineage ALL (about 15–20 percent), some follicular lymphomas and multiple myeloma cells (weaker expression) (see Fig. 4.2)
	anti-immunoglobulin*	immunoglobulin: as a surface membrane antigen in B cells (SmIg)
	anti-γ,α,μ,δ*	immunoglobulin heavy chains: cytoplasmic antigen in pre-B cells (Cy μ chain) and in late B lymphocytes and plasma cells
	anti-κ,λ*	immunoglobulin light chains: surface membrane antigen in B lymphocytes and cytoplasmic antigen in late B lymphocytes and plasma cells

*some antibodies in current use are polyclonal

Fig. 3.1 Monoclonal antibodies useful in the diagnosis and classification of acute leukaemia – those identifying mainly early precursor cells and cells of B-lineage.

Immunological markers in acute lymphoblastic leukaemia

Immunological markers separate ALL into leukaemias of B and T lineage. A useful panel of McAb for the detection of B-lineage blasts is CD19 and either CD22 (used in a method which allows detection of cytoplasmic antigen), CD20 or CD24. For T-lineage blasts a useful panel is CD7 (also reactive with some AML) and either CD3 (with the use of a technique for detection of cytoplasmic antigen), CD2 or CD5. The use of a wider panel of antibodies allows further separation into groups which are believed to reflect the normal maturation within these lineages.

MONOCLONAL ANTIBODIES USEFUL IN THE DIAGNOSIS AND CLASSIFICATION OF ACUTE LEUKAEMIA – THOSE IDENTIFYING MAINLY CELLS OF T LINEAGE

Cluster of differentiation	Representative McAb	Specificity within haemopoietic lineage
CD7	OKT16, Leu 9, 3A1, WT1	thymocytes, majority of mature T lymphocytes, NK cells, T- lineage ALL, 5–15 percent of AML, some leukaemias of mature T cells (see Fig. 4.15)
CD5	OKT1, OKT101, Leu 1, UCHT2	common and late thymocytes, some early thymocytes, T lymphocytes, T-lineage ALL, small subset of B lymphocytes, some leukaemias and lymphomas of mature B cells and mature T cells (see Figs. 4.2 and 4.15)
CD2	OKT11, Leu 5	E receptor, ligand for LFA-3: common and late thymocytes, mature T lymphocytes, about 80 percent of T-lineage ALL, leukaemias of mature T cells
CD1	OKT6, Leu 6	common thymocytes, some T-lineage ALL
CD4	OKT4, Leu 3a	common thymocytes (coexpressed with CD8), late thymocytes, subset of mature T cells, some leukaemias of mature T cells (see Fig. 4.15), monocytes
CD8	OKT8, Leu 2a	common thymocytes (coexpressed with CD4), late thymocytes, subset of mature T cells, some leukaemias of mature T cells (see Fig. 4.15)
CD3	OKT3, UCHT1, Leu 4	linked to T receptor: membrane antigen in late thymocytes and mature T lymphocytes, in about 25 percent of T-lineage ALL and in leukaemias of mature T cells; cytoplasmic antigen in the majority of thymocytes, and in almost all T-lineage ALL

Fig. 3.2 Monoclonal antibodies useful in the diagnosis and classification of acute leukaemia – those identifying mainly cells of T-lineage.

Study of CD10 (the CALLA or common ALL antigen), cytoplasmic immunoglobulin (μ chain, CyIg) and surface immunoglobulin (SmIg) allows B-lineage ALL to be separated into early B-precursor ALL, common ALL, pre-B ALL (CyIg positive) and B-ALL (SmIg positive) (Fig. 3.3). This classification implies that cases of B-lineage ALL which are CD10 negative and lack CyIg and SmIg represent an early stage of B-lymphocyte development. This view is widely accepted but it has been pointed out that CD10 negativity does not in fact correlate with markers of cellular immaturity and may actually represent an abnormal rather than an immature phenotype[5]. The term common ALL was initially used to designate all cases which showed the common ALL antigen. Since CyIg has been increasingly studied, pre-B cases have sometimes been included in the common ALL category and sometimes excluded. The MIC group has suggested that pre-B ALL should constitute a separate category[3] (Fig. 3.3). This categorization can be justified since pre-B cases have been found to have a worse prognosis than other non-B, non-T-lineage ALL[10], but it requires that CyIg be consistently studied or pre-B cases will be inadvertently grouped with common ALL.

Immunophenotyping of T-lineage ALL permits recognition of T-cell and precursor-T phenotype. A cell can be classified as a T cell when it forms E-rosettes or when the CD2 antigen is detectable; however, although the CD2 McAb detects the antigen which is responsible for E-rosetting, the concordance between these two criteria is far from perfect[7]. The MIC group[3] have suggested that classification be on the basis of either E-rosetting or CD2 reactivity, with early T-precursor ALL being

A MORPHOLOGICAL, IMMUNOLOGICAL AND CYTOGENETIC CLASSIFICATION OF ACUTE LYMPHOBLASTIC LEUKAEMIA OF B LINEAGE[3]

Category and karyotype*		Cell markers						FAB morphology	Percentage of cases of B-lineage ALL
		TdT	Ia	CD19	CD10	CyIg	SmIg		
Early B-precursor ALL	t(4;11) t(9;22) (Ph pos)	POS	POS	POS	NEG	NEG	NEG	L1 or L2	7–10
common ALL	6q− near haploid** t or del (12p) t(9;22) (Ph pos) 9p− hyperdiploid† tdic(9;12)[9]	POS	POS	POS	POS	NEG	NEG	L1 or L2	≃70
pre-B ALL	t(1;19)*** t(9;22) (Ph pos) 6q− hyperdiploid† translocations also associated with Burkitt's lymphoma (see below)	POS	POS	POS	POS	POS	NEG	L1 or L2	≃20
B-cell ALL	translocations also associated with Burkitt's lymphoma: t(8;14) t(8;22) t(2;8) 6q− 12p12 breakpoint	NEG	POS	POS	POS OR NEG	NEG OR POS	POS	L3	1–2

Precursor B-ALL CD22+

* the associations between immunological category and karyotype are characteristic but not exclusive
** mainly L2
*** mainly L1
† hyperdiploid with more than 50 chromosomes[8]

dic = dicentric
t = translocation

Fig. 3.3 A morphological, immunological and cytogenetic (MIC) classification of B-lineage ALL – expanded and modified from reference 3. TdT, Ia, CD19, CD10, CyIg (Cy μ chain) and SmIg as defined in Fig. 3.1.

CD7+CD2/ERFC− and T-cell ALL being CD7+CD2/ERFC+ (Fig. 3.4). Others have divided T-lineage ALL into three groups on the basis of CD1 and membrane CD3 reactivity[11] and have found that in children an early thymocyte phenotype (CD7+CD2+CD1−CD3−) was associated with an appreciably lower remission rate than was found in cases with an intermediate (CD7+CD2+CD1+CD3−) or mature (CD7+CD2+CD1−CD3+) thymocyte phenotype. In another study of adults classified on the basis of ERFC those who were ERFC− were found to have a prethymic phenotype (CD7+; CD1, CD4 and CD8−; CD2, CD3, CD10, Ia and CD34 variable) and a worse prognosis than ERFC+ cases[7]. The latter group could be divided into thymocytic phenotype

A MORPHOLOGICAL, IMMUNOLOGICAL AND CYTOGENETIC CLASSIFICATION OF ACUTE LYMPHOBLASTIC LEUKAEMIA OF T LINEAGE[3]						
Category and karyotype*		Cell markers			FAB morphology	Percentage of T-lineage ALL
		TdT	CD7	E-receptor or CD2		
Early T-precursor ALL	t or del 9p	POS	POS	NEG	LI or L2	≈30
T-cell ALL	t(11;14) 6q−	POS	POS	POS	LI or L2	≈70
*the associations between immunological category and karyotype are characteristic but not exclusive						

Fig. 3.4 A morphological, immunological and cytogenetic (MIC) classification of T-lineage ALL – modified from reference 3. E receptor = receptor for sheep red blood cells; TdT, CD7 and CD2 as defined in Figs. 3.1 and 3.2.

(CD1+) and mature T-cell phenotype (CD1−) but these two groups did not differ in clinical features or prognosis. Although these and other studies have shown a relationship between phenotype and disease characteristics, there is not as yet consensus as to the optimal basis for further classification of T-lineage ALL. This is in part due to the heterogeneity of antigen expression. When cases of T-lineage ALL express CD10 the expression is weaker than in B-lineage ALL.

Immunological markers in acute myeloid leukaemia

Immunological markers which identify AML and distinguish it from ALL include reactivity with antibodies of the CD13, CD33 and CDw65 clusters and reactivity with a McAb such as MA1 which recognizes the MPO protein, including its proenzyme form[12] (Fig. 3.5). CD13 is most sensitive when used with a technique which allows cytoplasmic antigen to be detected, since the antigen appears earlier in the cytoplasm than on the cell membrane[13]. The same groups of antibodies can be used for the diagnosis of AML M0.

The use of a wider panel of McAb shows different patterns of reactivity within the different FAB classes, although the correlation is not very tight (Fig. 3.6). CD13, CD33, CDw65 and MA1 show little difference between the FAB classes while other McAb show some selectivity for immature cells, for more mature cells, for granulocytic differentiation or for monocytic differentiation.

TdT and CD34 are markers of haemopoietic precursor cells of various lineages; among cases of AML, positivity is largely confined to the immature leukaemic cells of M0 and M1 AML[16]. HLA-Dr (Ia) is also expressed on haemopoietic precursor cells but continues to be expressed up to the myeloblast stage in granulocytic maturation and up to the mature monocyte in monocyte maturation. It is, therefore, widely expressed among cases of AML but is generally negative in AML M3.

CD13, CD33 and CD15 antibodies give positive reactions with leukaemic cells showing evidence of myeloid differentiation. Of these three specificities CD13 antibodies react with the majority of cases of M1–M5 AML though with a somewhat lower percentage of cases being positive when there is monocytic differentiation (M4 and M5); CD13 also gives positive reactions in the least mature leukaemias (M0). CD33 antibodies are less likely to react with M0 AML but reactions are generally positive in M1–M5. CD15 antibodies are generally negative in M1 AML but are positive in M2, M4 and M5b[2,17]; reactions in AML M3 and M5a are less consistent. Despite the mainly negative reactions in M1, one CD15 McAb was found to give positive reactions in more than 50 percent of M0 AML[19].

MONOCLONAL ANTIBODIES USEFUL IN THE DIAGNOSIS AND CLASSIFICATION OF ACUTE LEUKAEMIA – McAb IDENTIFYING MAINLY MYELOID CELLS

Cluster of differentiation	Representative McAb	Specificity within haemopoietic lineage
CD13	My 7, MCS.2	pan-myeloid: about 80 percent of AML (higher if sought as cytoplasmic antigen)[13], about 10 percent of B-lineage ALL[5]
CD33	My9, L4F3	myeloid progenitors and some maturing myeloid cells (myeloblasts, promyelocytes, myelocytes, monocytes), about 80 percent of AML, about 10 percent of B-lineage ALL[5]
CD15	Leu M1, MCS.1, FMC10, VIM D5	maturing myeloid cells (granulocytic more than monocytic), hairy cells
CD11b	Mo1, OKM1, Leu 15	C3bi receptor: mature monocytes, most monocytic and some granulocytic leukaemias, NK cells
CD14	My4, Mo2, UCHM1, FMC17, Leu M3	monocytes, macrophages, monocytic and some granulocytic leukaemias
CDw65	VIM2	granulocytic and monocytic lineages
CD41	J15	platelet glycoprotein IIb/IIIa complex (CD41a) and platelet glycoprotein IIb (CD41b): megakaryoblasts, megakaryocytes, platelets
CD42a	FMC25, BL-H6	platelet glycoprotein IX: megakaryoblasts, megakaryocytes
CD42b	AN51	platelet glycoprotein Ib: platelets
CD61	C15, C17	platelet glycoprotein IIIa
CD36	FA6–152, OKM5, 5F1	erythroblasts and progenitors, monocytes, macrophages, megakaryoblasts, megakaryocytes and platelets (platelet glycoprotein IV)
CD71	OKT9	transferrin receptor: erythroid cells, immature thymocytes, T-lineage ALL
unclustered	LICR-LON, R-10, R18, R23, VIE G4	glycophorin A: erythroid cells
unclustered	MA1	myeloperoxidase: myeloid cells (granulocytic more than monocytic)

Fig. 3.5 Monoclonal antibodies useful in the diagnosis and classification of acute leukaemia – those identifying mainly myeloid cells.

PATTERN OF REACTIVITY WITH MONOCLONAL ANTIBODIES COMMONLY OBSERVED IN FAB CATEGORIES OF AML									
	Markers of precursor cells			**Myeloid markers**			**Monocyte markers**		**Other**
	TdT*	Ia** (HLA DR)	CD34*** (3C5, My10)	CD13 (My7, MCS-2)	CD33 (My9, L4F3)	CD15 (Leu M1, VIM-D5, FMC10)	CD11b (Mo1, OKM1)	CD14 (UCHM1, My4, Mo2, Leu M3)	
M0	POS or NEG	POS	POS	MAINLY POS	POS or NEG	POS or NEG	MAINLY NEG	MAINLY NEG	
M1	POS or NEG	POS	MAINLY POS	MAINLY POS	POS	MAINLY NEG	POS or NEG	MAINLY NEG	
M2	NEG	POS	MAINLY NEG	POS	POS	POS	POS or NEG	MAINLY NEG	granulocyte markers†
M3	NEG	NEG	NEG	POS	POS	POS or NEG	MAINLY NEG	MAINLY NEG	granulocyte markers†
M4	NEG	POS	MAINLY NEG	MAINLY POS	POS	POS	POS	POS	other monocyte markers‡
M5	NEG	POS	MAINLY NEG	POS or NEG	POS	POS	POS	POS	other monocyte markers‡
M6	NEG	POS or NEG	NEG	POS or NEG	POS or NEG	MAINLY NEG	POS or NEG	MAINLY NEG	glycophorin A
M7	NEG	MAINLY POS	MAINLY POS	MAINLY NEG	POS or NEG	NEG	NEG	NEG	platelet glycoproteins
Overall AML	MAINLY NEG (10–20% pos)	POS (about 70%)	NEG or POS (about 30–40% pos)	POS (60–90%)	POS (70–90%)	POS (40–70%)	POS (50–60%)	NEG or POS (about 40% pos)	

* also positive in ALL with the exception of the minority of cases with mature-B phenotype
** also positive in ALL of B-lineage and in occasional cases of T-lineage ALL
*** also positive in some B-lineage ALL but not mature B-ALL
† e.g. PMN 81, PMN 29[14]
‡ e.g. UCALF[15]

Fig. 3.6 The pattern of reactivity with monoclonal antibodies most commonly observed in the FAB subtypes of AML. Markers as defined in Figs. 3.1 and 3.5. Derived from references 2, 14–20 and other sources.

CD11b and CD14 antibodies show some specificity for leukaemias with monocytic differentiation. CD14 antibodies are superior to CD11b antibodies for distinguishing M4 and M5 AML from M1, M2 and M3 AML[15,16,17]. UCHALF (reactive with surface-bound lactoferrin) has also been found to be a sensitive and specific indicator of monocytic differentiation[15]. M5a and M5b show some differences in their patterns of reaction with McAb. The less mature cells of M5a are more likely to give negative reactions with antibodies of CD13, CD15, CD11b and CD14 clusters[17].

M3 and M3V show a characteristic pattern of reaction with McAb which may be of diagnostic importance in distinguishing between M3V and M5 AML. M3 and its variant are usually negative for both Ia and CD34, these being markers which are positive on early granulocytic cells but become negative by the promyelocyte stage. CD13 and CD33 are characteristically positive. CD9 is almost always positive, whereas it is negative in most other FAB subtypes of AML. M3 and M3V share with M2 a high rate of positivity with McAb reactive with mature granulocytes. Positive reactions sometimes occur with CD11b and CD14 McAb; these reactions, more typical of monocytes, do not correlate with anomalous expression of nonspecific esterase by M3 cells[21].

Immunological markers are important in the diagnosis of AML M7 since they are more specific than cytochemistry and more widely available than the PPO reaction which requires ultrastructural cytochemistry for its detection. The usual order of appearance of markers in the megakaryocyte lineage is probably Ia, PPO and acid phosphatase followed by CD33, CD34 and ANAE activity, followed in turn by platelet glycoprotein IIIa (CD61), glycoprotein IIb and the IIb/IIIa complex (CD41), glycoprotein IX and Ib (CD42a and b), and finally the Von Willebrand antigen (best detected by polyclonal antibodies) and PAS positivity. CD41 (J15) and CD61 McAb (C15, C17) have some advantages over CD42 McAb (AN51); they are more sensitive since the antigen appears earlier, and also more specific since occasional cases of ALL and AML M5 have been found to be positive with CD42 McAb[22]. Reactivity with myeloid McAb CD33 and CD34 is seen only in early cells in the megakaryocyte lineage, in megakaryoblasts and immature megakaryocytes.

Diagnosis of AML M6, particularly when the cells have a very immature phenotype, is aided by the use of immunological markers[23]. The earliest recognizable erythroid cells have a number of markers which are not specific to this lineage including Ia, the transferrin receptor (CD71), certain blood group antigens (A, B and H; I and i) and reactivity with the McAb FA6.152 (CD36). Although not specific, CD71 reactivity is suggestive of erythroid differentiation since it is rarely present in other myeloid leukaemias. CD36 McAb, however, react also with megakaryoblasts[24]. The earliest specific erythroid markers are carbonic anhydrase I activity, detectable by a polyclonal antibody[23] and reactivity with the McAb EP-1[25], followed shortly after by reactivity with the McAb SFL23.6[25]. Spectrin (detectable by a polyclonal antibody) and glycophorin A appear later, in the case of normal erythroid development shortly before the appearance of haemoglobin. The gero McAb which recognizes the Gerbich blood group antigen is also useful in the diagnosis of M6.

Bilineage and biphenotypic leukaemias

Terminology in this area is very confused. The word 'bilineage' is usually used to indicate that some leukaemic cells are myeloid and others are lymphoid; the designation 'biclonal' is better avoided since two apparently distinct leukaemic populations may actually derive from one aberrant stem cell. The term biphenotypic indicates that there are leukaemic cells with phenotypic characteristics of both lymphoid and myeloid cells; 'hybrid' and 'mixed-lineage' have been used similarly. It may be inferred that a leukaemia is biphenotypic if the percentage of cells having myeloid markers overlaps with the percentage of cells having lymphoid markers, but the diagnosis is more firmly based if a double labelling technique is employed, combining two immunological markers or cytochemistry and an immunological marker. Bilineage leukaemia, and sometimes biphenotypic leukaemias, can be suspected on morphological grounds when blasts appear to be of two distinct types. However, in general, immunological markers are needed to define a bilineage or biphenotypic leukaemia since there are few morphological or cytochemical features which can be considered to prove that a cell is lymphoid. Acceptable evidence for myeloid differentiation includes the presence of Auer rods, a positive cytochemical reaction for MPO or CAE, or a strong diffuse reaction for nonspecific esterase, but in the context of a suspected bilineage or biphenotypic leukaemia, SBB positivity alone should probably not be regarded as a myeloid marker since occasional cases of apparent lymphoblastic leukaemia have given positive reactions. Similarly, immunological markers are generally lineage-associated rather than lineage-specific and several, including CD7 and TdT, are not infrequently expressed in an 'inappropriate' lineage. del Vecchio et al.[6] employed a panel of 10 well characterized markers and found that 74 percent of 163 cases of acute leukaemia expressed only 'appropriate' markers. They suggested that the 18 percent of cases which expressed a single 'inappropriate' marker should be regarded as showing ectopic expression of an antigen and only the 5.5 percent which expressed two or more 'inappropriate' markers should be regarded as biphenotypic leukaemia. Mirro and Kitchingman[26] proposed a more comprehensive scheme in which morphologic, cytochemical, immunological and karyotypic features were weighted according to the strength of their association with one or other lineage, with a minimum score of 1 for each lineage being required for a leukaemia to be classified as mixed-lineage; in this scheme also the expression of a single 'inappropriate' antigen is not sufficient to establish a lineage.

CYTOGENETIC ABNORMALITIES AND THE FAB SUBTYPES OF ACUTE LEUKAEMIA

In both acute leukaemia and the MDS normal polyclonal haemopoietic cells are largely replaced by abnormal cells which are the progeny of a single cell and are therefore designated a clone. In AML the abnormal clone of cells may include the granulocyte/monocyte, erythroid and megakaryocyte lineages or be restricted to the granulocytic/monocytic lineage.

In many instances the abnormal clone of cells has an acquired chromosomal abnormality which can be detected by examination of the chromosomes of cells arrested in metaphase. The bone marrow cells may be examined directly or after a period in culture with or without various mitogens and synchronizing agents. All of a population of leukaemic cells may show the same chromosomal abnormality, or further clonal evolution may have occurred so that some cells have a further abnormality and represent a daughter clone or subclone. In cytogenetic terminology they are sublines or sidelines derived from the stemline. Residual normal haemopoietic cells are karyotypically normal unless the patient happens to have a constitutional chromosome abnormality. When the bone marrow cells of a patient with acute leukaemia are examined they may be found to be all karyotypically abnormal (AA) or all karyotypically normal (NN), or there may be a mixture of normal and abnormal metaphases (AN). The latter situation almost always represents a mixture of normal and leukaemic cells. The presence of only normal metaphases may be because the leukaemic clone does not have a chromosomal abnormality detectable by microscopy or may indicate that only normal cells are entering mitosis in vitro. The initial failure of some centres to detect the characteristic chromosomal abnormality of AML M3 was subsequently found to be due to the use of a technique of direct examination so that only karyotypically normal erythroid cells were in mitosis[27,28], M3 being one of the types of leukaemia in which the erythroid and megakaryocyte lineages are not part of the leukaemic clone. Other centres where cells were cultured before examination detected the characteristic abnormality because the culture conditions selected for leukaemic cells.

Occasionally karyotypic evidence suggests the presence of two independent clones. Although this does occur, particularly when a bone marrow has been exposed to mutagenic influences, evidence from G6PD alloenzymes suggests that in some patients apparently independent clones are daughter clones derived from a cytogenetically normal parent clone. Similarly, a mixture of normal and abnormal metaphases can be consequent on a cytogenetic abnormality being present only in a daughter clone.

When the karyotype of bone marrow cells is studied some cells show random abnormalities which need to be distinguished from a nonrandom or consistent abnormality which indicates the presence of an abnormal clone. For this reason a clone is considered to be present if two cells show the same structural change or additional chromosomes, or if three cells show the same missing chromosome[29]. Various terms and abbreviations which are used in describing chromosomes and their abnormalities are shown in Fig. 3.7. Translocations are described as reciprocal if material is exchanged between chromosomes and as nonreciprocal when materaial from one chromosome is transferred to another. A balanced translocation is one in which there is no net gain or loss of chromosomal material, whereas an unbalanced translocation is one in which translocation is associated with loss or duplication of all or part of a chromosome. Translocations are described in a shorthand manner as follows:- t(15;17)(q22;q12) indicates that there is a reciprocal translocation between chromosomes 15 and 17; the breakpoints are at band q22 on chromosome 15 and at band q12 on chromosome 17. This is the translocation found in M3 and M3V, the first specific abnormality to be linked to a morphologically recognizable subtype of acute leukaemia. When describing trans-

ABBREVIATIONS AND TERMINOLOGY USED IN DESCRIBING CHROMOSOMES AND THEIR ABNORMALITIES	
p	short arm of a chromosome
q	long arm of a chromosome
p+, q+	addition of chromosomal material to the short arm or long arm respectively
p−, q−	loss of chromosomal material from the short arm or long arm respectively
del	deletion
der	derivative chromosome (a derivative chromosome is an abnormal chromosome derived from two or more chromosomes; it takes its number from the chromosome which contributes the centromere)
dic	dicentric (a chromosome with two centromeres)
dm	double minute (see minute)
inv	inversion
ins	insertion [may be direct (dir) or inverted (inv)]
iso	isochromosome (a chromosome formed by duplication of the long arm or the short arm)
mar	marker chromosome (an abnormal chromosome which is not fully characterized)
min	minute (an acentric fragment smaller than the width of a single chromatid; may be single or double)
r	ring chromosome
t	translocation
+	addition of a chromosome
−	loss of a chromosome
aneuploid	cells having an abnormal number of chromosomes which is neither half nor a multiple of 46
diploid	cells having the normal complement of 46 chromosomes (23 pairs)
haploid	cells with 23 (unpaired) chromosomes
pseudo-diploid	cells having 46 chromosomes but with structural abnormalities being present
tetraploid	cells having 92 chromosomes (four sets)
karyotype	systematized array of the chromosomes of a cell and by extension of a clone of cells (or an individual)
centromere	the junction of the short arm (p) and the long arm (q)
paracentric inversion	inversion of a segment of a chromosome confined to one arm
pericentric inversion	inversion of a segment of a chromosome composed of part of both arms and the centromere

Fig. 3.7 Terminology and abbreviations used in describing chromosomes and their abnormalities.

locations the chromosomes are listed in numerical order. When describing insertions, the chromosome into which material is inserted is listed first followed by the chromosome from which material has been derived.

Cytogenetic abnormalities and the MIC classification of acute lymphoblastic leukaemia

With techniques now available 70–90 percent of ALL cases have a demonstrable cytogenetic abnormality. The MIC classification[3] (Figs. 3.3 and 3.4) integrates morphology, immunophenotype and cytogenetics so that a case might be classified, for example, as early T-precursor/9p–/L2 or as B cell/t(8;14)/L3. The classification is open-ended so that new categories can be added as recognized.

Specific cytogenetic abnormalities can be related to the immunophenotype but, with the exception of the translocations characteristic of L3 ALL, they do not show a close relationship to the FAB subtype. Some cytogenetic abnormalities (such as 6q– and 9p–) are associated with both B- and T-lineage ALL[30,31], while others are confined to B-lineage or T-lineage ALL or are associated with specific phenotypes. Hyperdiploidy with a modal chromosome number of 47–50 or >50 is commonly associated with B-lineage ALL but is rare in T-lineage ALL[8,30], whereas translocations with breakpoints at the site of the T-cell receptor (TCR) α or β genes are largely confined to T-lineage ALL[30]. The translocations which are characteristic of Burkitt's lymphoma with breakpoints involving immunoglobulin genes are found in B-lineage ALL but not in T-lineage ALL; they occur most commonly, but not exclusively, in B-cell/L3 ALL. As in the case of Burkitt's lymphoma, t(8;14)(q24;q32) is by far the commonest abnormality, followed by t(8;22)(q24;q11) and t(2;8)(p11.2;q24). Translocations with a 12p12 breakpoint including t(7;12)(q11;p12) and t(dic)(9;12)(p11;p12) have recently been found to be associated with B-lineage ALL[9,31]. The t(1;19)(q23;p13) translocation is strongly associated with pre-B ALL, usually with L1 morphology. There is a similar strong association between t(4;11)(q21;q23) and early B-precursor ALL, although occasional cases are common ALL or pre-B ALL and the morphology may be either L1 or L2. The t(4;11) translocation is particularly common among cases of congenital ALL and ALL in young infants. These cases are also characterized by marked splenomegaly and a high white cell count[32]. It is probable that

the 11q23 breakpoint is critical in the association with early precursor-B ALL since the same immunophenotype has also been associated with other translocations involving this breakpoint, including t(9;11)[33], t(11;17)[34] and t(11;19)[33].

In T-lineage ALL there is also some correlation between immunological phenotype and specific cytogenetic abnormalities although neither correlates with the FAB type (Fig. 3.4). About one-quarter of cases of T-lineage ALL are associated with a variety of translocations, all of which involve genes which are important in T-cell function, particularly the TCR α and δ genes at 14q11–13, the TCR β gene at 7q32–36[30] and occasionally the TCR γ gene at 7p13. Examples of such translocations are t(11;14)(p13;q11–13) and t(7;14)(q35;q11).

In ALL, chromosomal abnormalities correlate with other clinical and haematological factors of prognostic importance but they also have an independent prognostic significance, particularly in children[35,36,37]. The translocations associated with Burkitt's lymphoma, and also t(1;19), t(4;11) and t(9;22) (with formation of the Philadelphia chromosome), indicate a very poor prognosis. Whether other pseudodiploid cases have an equally poor prognosis is disputed[35,37,38]. The best prognosis is associated with hyperdiploidy with a modal chromosome number of more than 50 and with a normal karyotype, while 6q– cases are intermediate.

Cytogenetic abnormalities and the MIC classification of acute myeloid leukaemia

With current techniques 70–85 percent[39] of patients with AML are found to have nonrandom (clonal) cytogenetic abnormalities, many of which are recurrent. Overall the commonest cytogenetic abnormality is trisomy 8, with anomalies of chromosome 7 in second place. Some chromosomal anomalies, such as trisomy 8 and trisomy 21, are found in all FAB subtypes and in both secondary and *de novo* leukaemia; they are not related to any readily apparent morphological or clinical features. Other anomalies, including t(15;17), t(8;21) and t or inv(16), have a strong association with a particular FAB type and are associated with specific morphological features; they rarely, if ever, occur in secondary leukaemia, and dysplasia of erythroid and megakaryocyte lineages is not usually a feature. It is possible that in this group of anomalies the leukaemia has arisen in a lineage-restricted stem cell. Other anomalies such as t(6;9), t(1;7), t(3;3) and inv(3) occur in multiple FAB subtypes and in myelodysplasia, as well as in both *de novo* and secondary (irradiation or cytotoxic drug related) leukaemias; it is likely that the association of such translocations with bi or trilineage myelodysplasia and with multiple FAB categories indicates that the leukaemia has arisen in a multipotent stem cell which has preserved its capacity to differentiate in various directions. Other anomalies which involve predominantly loss of chromosomal material (such as -5, $5q-$, -7, $7q-$) show a similar lack of relationship to FAB types, but an association with myelodysplastic features and with therapy-related MDS and secondary AML. Many patients with AML have more than one karyotypic abnormality. Complex abnormalities are particularly characteristic of M6 AML, secondary AML and AML arising in patients with MDS. Chromosomal abnormalities which are strongly associated with characteristic clinical and morphological features are often termed 'specific' whereas those which are not are termed nonspecific.

Chromosomal abnormalities have been found to have independent prognostic significance in AML although the prognostic ranking has not been identical in different series of patients[39,40,41,42]. In general, the best prognosis is seen with inv(16) and the worst with deletions or monosomies of chromosomes 5, 7 or both, t(1;7), t(6;9), inv(3), t(3;3) and complex karyotypic abnormalities. An intermediate prognosis is seen with t(8;21), t(15;17), and translocations involving 11q23.

The MIC Cooperative Study Group[4] proposed that cases of AML should be studied by morphological, immunological and cytogenetic techniques. They defined 10 categories, but the classification is open-ended and new categories can be added once they have been clearly defined. Subtypes of leukaemia based on categorization by morphology and cytogenetics according to the MIC system will now be described.

M2/t(8;21)

One of the two commonest specific translocations in AML is t(8;21)(q22;q22)[43,44,45,46] (Fig. 3.8), the other being t(15;17). The t(8;21) translocation is strongly associated with M2 AML, with a minority of cases being M1 or M4. Overall, cases of M2/t(8;21) comprise about 9 percent of AML[47]; cases are relatively more common in children (14 percent of AML) than in adults (6 percent of AML). Adult cases are usually young and more often male than female. The geographical distribution appears to be uneven with a higher percentage of cases showing this abnormality in Japan, among non-Whites in South Africa[45] and in China[48]. M2/t(8;21) is very rare in secondary leukaemia[45]. In some studies of patients with M2/t(8;21), median survival has been longer than the average for AML but in other studies this has not been so, particularly when comparison has been made with age-matched controls. Formation of solid tumours of leukaemic cells is not uncommon.

Variant karyotypic abnormalities which may be associated with this subtype of AML include del(8)(q22) and complex translocations involving a third chromosome together with 8 and 21. Common associated karyotypic abnormalities are loss of the Y chromosome in males or loss of the inactive X chromosome in females. A less frequent nonrandom association is 9q− consequent on an interstitial deletion.

Characteristic morphological features are observed[46] (Figs. 3.9–3.11, see also Fig. 1.3). There is maturation of leukaemic cells to neutrophils and consequently severe neutropenia is uncommon and some patients have neutrophilia. The blasts are very heterogeneous, variable in size but often large and with a high nucleocytoplasmic ratio. Nuclei are commonly indented or cleft with large nucleoli. Cytoplasm may be basophilic (Fig. 3.9b), sometimes vacuolated. In more mature cells basophilia is sometimes confined to the periphery of the cytoplasm (Fig. 3.9c). Auer rods are common, with often a single slender Auer rod per cell. Some blasts may contain giant granules, as may maturing cells. Binucleated myeloblasts, promyeloblasts, myelocytes and metamyelocytes are seen[43]. Maturing cells of the granulocytic series show Auer rods which may be found even in neutrophils. Hypogranularity, bizarre-shaped nuclei and the acquired Pelger–Huët anomaly are also present in neutrophils. Bone marrow eosinophilia occurs in a proportion of patients who may be classified as having M2Eo. Some of the bone marrow eosinophils may have basophilic granules but this feature is much less marked than in inv(16)/M4Eo (see below)[44]. Most patients do not have a peripheral blood eosinophilia but occasional patients have had a markedly elevated eosinophil count[49,50], sometimes with an associated hypereosinophilic syndrome[50]. Myelodysplastic features in erythroid and megakaryocyte lineages are not usually seen. Eosinophils can be demonstrated to be part of the cytogenetically abnormal clone whereas the erythroid[44] and megakaryocyte lineages probably are not.

Cytochemical stains[46,51] show localized SBB and MPO positivity in the blasts, often confined to the

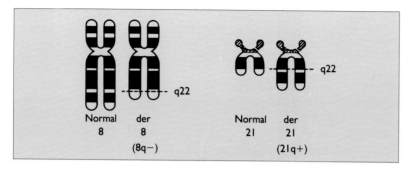

Fig. 3.8 A diagrammatic representation of the t(8;21)(q22;q22) abnormality. The breakpoints in the two derivative chromosomes are indicated. Modified from reference 4.

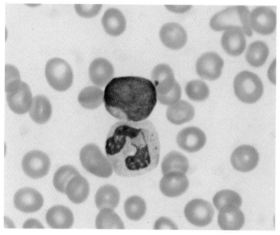

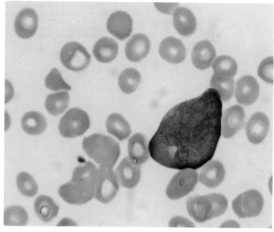

Fig. 3.9 PB and BM films of a patient with M2/t(8;21). **(a)** PB stained with MGG showing a blast cell and an abnormal neutrophil. × 960.

(b) PB stained with MGG showing a strongly basophilic blast with a paranuclear indentation representing the Golgi zone. × 960.

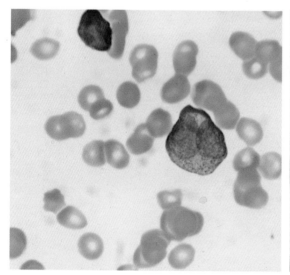

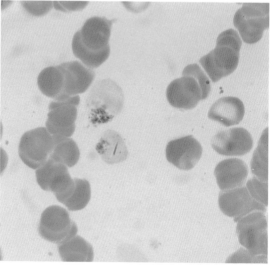

(c) PB stained with MGG showing an abnormal promyelocyte with peripheral basophilia. × 960.

(d) BM stained for peroxidase activity showing two blasts with positive granules in the indentation of the nucleus. One blast also contains an Auer rod. × 960.

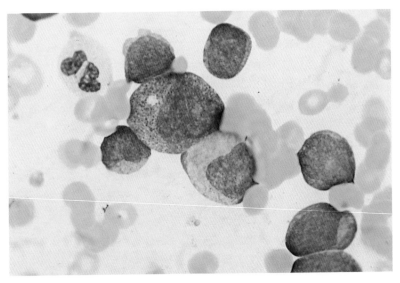

Fig. 3.10 BM of a patient with M2/t(8;21) showing blasts and maturing granulocytic cells including a hypogranular neutrophil. MGG × 960.

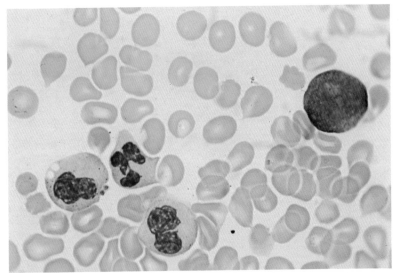

Fig. 3.11 BM of a patient with M2/t(8;21).
(a) MGG stain showing a blast and three abnormal neutrophils. × 960.

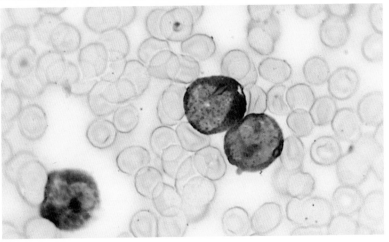

(b) SBB stain showing strongly positive cells in one of which an Auer rod with a hollow core can be seen. × 960.

indentation of the nucleus (Fig. 3.9d). CAE is strongly positive. Cytochemical stains may show that Auer rods are in fact multiple, and occasionally they are revealed in eosinophils as well as in the neutrophil series; Auer rods are sometimes positive for CAE and PAS as well as for MPO and SBB. Auer rods may have a nonstaining core (Fig. 3.11b). The eosinophils in t(8;21)/M2 do not show the aberrant positivity for CAE which is a feature of inv(16)/M4Eo[44]. The NAP score is generally low[52], but neutrophils which are negative for SBB and MPO are uncommon[51]. Blasts are more commonly PAS positive than in AML in general; the pattern of staining is diffuse with some granules and rare blocks. PAS-positive erythroblasts are not a feature. Eosinophil granules may show aberrant PAS positivity[46].

M3 or M3V/t(15;17)

The t(15;17)(q22;q12 or 21) translocation (Fig. 3.12) is present in the great majority of patients with M3 and M3V AML and, with the exception of rare conditions such as hypergranular promyelocytic transformation of CGL, is confined to this category of leukaemia. Overall, M3/M3V/t(15;17) constitute about 9 percent of cases of AML[47]. In a minority of cases variant translocations occur which involve both chromosomes 15 and 17 and a third chromosome. Rare patients have been reported in whom there was a translocation or other abnormality of either chromosome 17 or, less often, chromosome 15 with no apparent abnormality of the other member of the pair. The frequency with which the specific t(15;17)

abnormality is detected is method-dependent, the apparent frequency increasing when the bone marrow is cultured rather than being examined directly, and increasing further when methotrexate synchronization is used[28]. This is the reason for the apparent geographic variation in the frequency of the translocation in cases of M3 AML which was previously reported. Nevertheless, some cases of M3 lack the t(15;17) abnormality but show another clonal karyotypic abnormality such as +8 or +21[47]. The most common associated karyotypic abnormalities are +8 and i(17q−).

The distinctive morphological and cytochemical features of this type of leukaemia have been described on page 13.

M5/del(11)(q23) or M5/t(11q)

There is a strong association between monoblastic/monocytic leukaemia and deletions or translocations involving band 23 of 11q[53]. The leukaemias have been mainly M5a but sometimes are M5b or M4 and occasionally M1 or M2. Auer rods are quite uncommon. Overall such cases comprise about 4 percent of AML[47]. The prevalence is highest among young infants and babies with congenital leukaemia but adult cases also occur. The prognosis has varied considerably between different series of patients. The deletions have been interpreted both as interstitial and terminal. Translocations have included t(9;11)(p21–22;q23), t(10;11)(p11–15;q23), t(11;17)(q23;q21–25), t(11;19)(q23;p13) and, less commonly, translocations between chromosome 11 and other

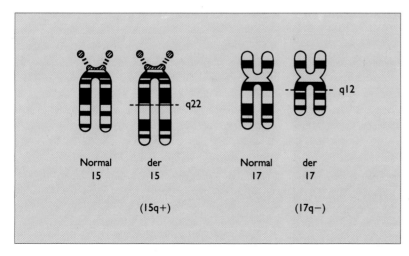

Fig. 3.12 A diagrammatic representation of the t(15;17)(q22;q12 or q21) abnormality. Modified from reference 4.

Normal 15   der 15   Normal 17   der 17

(15q+)   (17q−)

chromosomes including 1, 2, 5, 6, 11, 13 or 22. Some translocations with an 11q23 breakpoint, including the commonest t(9;11), are difficult to detect. Leukaemias in which there are deletions and translocations involving 11q14 are generally also M5a, M5b or M4.

There appears to be a subtle difference between t(4;11)(q21;q23) and the translocations listed above which share the 11q23 breakpoint. Although t(4;11) can be associated with M5a, it is not associated with M5b or M4 but rather with a group of leukaemias of very immature phenotype. These cases share common clinical and haematological features although the phenotype of the cells varies from monoblastic to early B-precursor or biphenotypic/bilineage leukaemias (see page 79). However other translocations with an 11q23 breakpoint have also been associated, although less frequently, with early B-precursor and biphenotypic/bilineage leukaemias so the difference is not clearcut.

M4Eo/inv(16)

Abnormalities of chromosome 16 band q22, particularly inversion 16 [inv(16)(p13;q22)] (Fig. 3.13), are associated with a subtype of M4 in which there is prominent proliferation of abnormal eosinophils (M4Eo)[54,28] (Fig. 3.14 and see also Fig. 1.21). Occasional cases are classified as M2Eo rather than M4Eo. The latter has also been described in association with a deletion [del(16)(q22)][55] and occasionally with translocations [for example t(16;16)(p13;q22) and t(5;16)(q33;q22)]. M4Eo with an abnormality of 16q22 comprises about 3 percent of AML cases. Both inv(16) and del(16) are relatively difficult to detect and it can also be difficult to distinguish between the various abnormalities of chromosome 16[28]. The commonest associated chromosomal abnormalities are trisomy 8, trisomy 22 and 7q−, the latter two anomalies being uncommon in association with other specific chromosomal aberrations. M4Eo is sometimes associated with meningeal leukaemia and with intracranial tumour formation by leukaemic cells. There have also been several reports of granulocytic sarcoma of the bowel occurring in advance of overt leukaemia. Patients are relatively young; remission rate is high and prognosis good.

Blast cells are variable in size and shape with prominent cytoplasmic basophilia. Some are monoblasts and some are primitive cells with occasional eosinophil granules. Auer rods are usually present although only in a minority of cells; they are sometimes present in mature neutrophils. Bone marrow eosinophils and, to a greater extent, eosinophil myelocytes show prominent basophilic granules (Fig. 3.14a,b). Mature eosinophils may be hypolobulated. In some cases the eosinophils have unusually large and folded nuclei. Eosinophils also show aberrant cytochemical reactions. Some have PAS-positive granules and some give positive reactions for CAE. PAS-positive granules are not specific for this subtype of leukaemia, nor in fact for leukaemic eosinophils as they may be observed in t(8;21)/M2[46] and sometimes in reactive eosinophilia[28]. Positivity for CAE may, however, indicate that eosinophils are part of a leukaemic process[28]. Despite the bone marrow eosinophilia, peripheral blood eosinophilia is unusual and peripheral blood eosinophils are usually morphologically normal. Cytogenetic analysis has confirmed that eosinophils are indeed part of the abnormal clone. Occasional patients with M4Eo/inv(16) have had increased bone marrow basophils and basophil precursors (confirmed by metachromasia with toluidine blue)[56] (see Fig. 1.21a,b). Dysplasia of erythroid and megakaryocyte lineages is not usually seen.

Occasional patients with the morphological features of M4/Eo have not had a detectable abnormality of chromosome 16 and others with inv(16)(p13;q22) have had M4 rather than M4Eo or M2Eo. Most cases with del(16)(q22) have been considered to show the same features as are seen with inv(16), but there have been reports suggesting that patients with del(16)(q22) have M4 AML without eosinophilia[28,57] and with a high incidence of preceding MDS[57].

M1/t(9;22)

The reciprocal translocation t(9;22)(q34;q11) leads to the formation of the Philadelphia chromosome, an abbreviated chromosome 22 to which a small part of chromosome 9 has been translocated. The Philadelphia chromosome was initially designated by the abbreviation (Ph[1]), but it has been suggested that it is now more appropriate to omit the superscript[58]. The Ph chromosome was the first specific karyotypic abnormality to be recognized in relation to a human malignancy when its most characteristic association with CGL was described. It is also associated with ALL and AML. Ph-positive cases comprise less than 1 percent of AML. Cases are usually M1 and less often M2 or M4. Some are M0 including M0Baso. MPO activity may be weak or absent[59,28]. Auer rods are uncommon. Basophilia may be present. The commonest associated chromosomal aberrations are −7, +Ph and +8.

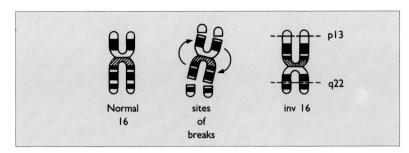

Fig. 3.13 A diagrammatic representation of inv(16)(p13;q22); this is an example of a pericentric inversion. Modified from reference 4.

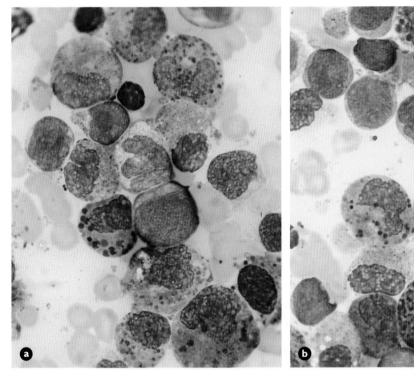

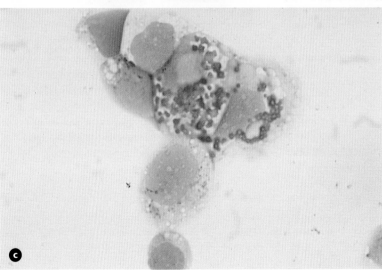

Fig. 3.14 BM of a patient with M4Eo/inv(16).
(a,b) MGG stain showing abnormal blasts, monocytes, mature eosinophils and eosinophil myelocytes with abnormal basophilic granules. × 960.
(c) SBB stain showing large abnormal granules in the eosinophil lineage and occasional small granules in monocytes. × 960.

M2 or M4Baso/t(6;9)

The t(6;9)(p23;q34.3) translocation[60,61,62] is associated with M2, less often M4 and least often with M1. This subtype comprises less than 1 percent of AML cases. The leukaemia may be secondary or develop *de novo*. Myelodysplastic features are quite common and a myelodysplastic syndrome may precede overt leukaemia. Bone marrow basophilia is common but not invariable and may also be present during the preceeding myelodysplasia[60]. The peripheral blood basophil count is also often elevated[60]. Some cases have also had increased bone marrow eosinophils. Auer rods are common[60,62]. Patients tend to be young but despite this the prognosis is poor[60,62]. It is likely that this leukaemia arises in a multipotent stem cell, often in a myelodysplastic setting.

The frequent association of this translocation with basophilia and the close similarity of the breakpoint on chromosome 9 to that in CGL led to speculation that the c-*abl* oncogene was implicated in the pathogenesis of this leukaemia. However the breakpoint is not identical to that in CGL[61] and in patients so far studied c-*abl* was neither translocated nor rearranged.

M1/inv(3)

Inv(3)(q21;q26) (Fig. 3.15) and related karyotypic abnormalities are associated with AML with a relative or absolute thrombocytosis, and with the bone marrow showing megakaryocytes which are morphologically abnormal and often also increased in number[63]. Such cases constitute less than 1 percent of AML[47]. Patients are usually elderly. The same chromosomal defect together with the megakaryocyte/platelet abnormality may be seen in the MDS (including RARS), in blast crisis of CGL, in AML evolving in the setting of the MDS, and in *de novo* and secondary AML.

The AML is most often M1 but cases can also be M2, M4, M6, M7 or unclassifiable. Trilineage myelodysplasia is usually prominent with hypogranular and pseudo-Pelger–Huët neutrophils, dyserythropoiesis including ring sideroblasts, giant and agranular platelets and abnormal megakaryocytes. The megakaryocytes are generally small with one or two small round nuclei (SRN megakaryocytes) or larger with a round nucleus (LRN megakaryocytes), but some patients have had multinucleated or unusually large megakaryocytes. Associated bone marrow fibrosis is sometimes present. Inv(3)(q21;q26) is the most common cytogenetic association with this type of leukaemia but other abnormalities involving the same two breakpoints have also been observed, including t(3;3)(q21;q26), ins(5;3)(q14;q21;q26) and ins(3;3)(q23 or 26;q21;q26). Morphologically similar cases have also been reported in which only the 3q21 breakpoint was involved, suggesting this may be the more critical of the two breakpoints; these variant karyotypic abnormalities have included t(1;3):p36;q21)[64], t(3;6)(q21;p21)[65] and del(3)(q12q21)[63].

The association of this related group of chromosomal anomalies with prominent trilineage myelodysplasia and with leukaemia of multiple FAB subtypes indicates that the leukaemia arises in a pluripotent stem cell, often in a myelodysplastic setting. The prognosis is poor.

M5/t(8;16)

The t(8;16)(p11;p13) translocation is associated with AML with monocytic differentiation. Such cases are rare, comprising less than 1 percent of AML[47]. More than half the reported cases have been M5, particularly M5a, with the majority of the remainder being M4. Many cases have been in infants and children. The majority of cases have shown haemophagocytosis by leukaemic cells, particularly erythrophagocytosis, to the extent that the first case was interpreted as malignant histiocytosis.

M2Baso/12p–

Deletions and translocations involving 12p band 11–13, such as del(12)(p11p13) (Fig. 3.16), are associated with AML M2 or M4 with basophilic differentiation. Such abnormalities occur in about 1.5 percent of AML cases[47]. The blasts of M2Baso cases may be difficult to recognize as myeloid by light microscopy alone since they are largely agranular; electron microscopy or the use of McAb may be necessary[4]. The blasts can also be identified by metachromatic staining with toluidine blue, Astra blue or SBB. M2Baso/12p– may occur as a secondary or a *de novo* AML. The same chromosomal defect is seen in MDS secondary to chemotherapy/radiotherapy.

M4/+4

Trisomy 4 is particularly associated with AML M4 and also with M1 or M2 AML. Such cases comprise well below 1 percent of AML cases.

M1/9q−

Del(9)(q13q22) is mainly associated with M1 AML[66]. Typical morphological features include a preponderance of agranular blasts with marked variation in size and a high nucleocytoplasmic ratio. The blasts commonly have Auer rods, vacuoles or both. Such cases are rare, comprising well below 1 percent of AML cases[47].

OTHER SUBTYPES

Other cytogenetic abnormalities, each of which is associated with fewer than 1 percent of AML cases, have been less well characterized. Possible new subtypes include M4/+22 and M2/t(7;11)(p15;p15)[67]. Other recurrent chromosomal abnormalities, including +11, i(17q), 20q−, t(3;5)(q25.1;q34)[68] and t(1;7)(p11;p11) have been associated with multiple FAB subtypes and often also with myelodysplastic features or preceding MDS, suggesting the abnormal clone has arisen from a multipotent stem cell.

Cytogenetic abnormalities and bilineage/biphenotypic leukaemia

L1 or L2/M5/t(4;11)

An association of t(4;11)(q21;q23) with ALL L1/L2 of an early B-precursor phenotype, with AML M5a and with bilineage/biphenotypic leukaemia has already been noted. In the biphenotypic/bilineage leukaemias the myeloid component is often of the monocytic lineage. Although the ALL component is usually early B-precursor, it is occasionally common or pre-B ALL. Some patients have either biphenotypic blasts or two blast populations at diagnosis, while others present with ALL and either have blasts of myeloid phenotype emerging early during the course of treatment or subsequently relapse with a myeloid phenotype.

Leukaemias with the t(4;11) abnormality can be seen as forming a single entity since they share clinical and haematological features[32]. About one-quarter of the cases described have been of congenital leukaemia and others have been in infants or young children, but cases also occur in adults. The leukaemia usually develops *de novo* although occasional cases have followed chemotherapy/radiotherapy[69]. At presentation, splenomegaly and hepatomegaly are often marked and the white cell count is usually high, sometimes very high[32]. The prognosis is poor, consequent on a relatively low complete remission rate together with a short remission duration.

Biphenotypic leukaemia has also been associated with other translocations and insertions which involve the 11q23 band, such as t(4;11;17)(q21;q23;q11)[70], ins(4;11)(q21;q23)[71], t(11;17)(q23;p13)[34], t(11;19)(q23;p13.3)[33] and t(9;11)(p22;q23)[33].

Other subtypes of biphenotypic leukaemia have been less well defined. Some cases have been associated with monosomy 7 and others with the Philadelphia chromosome.

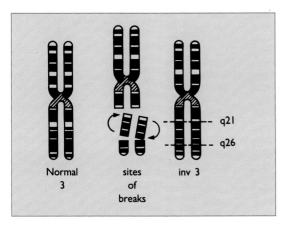

Fig. 3.15 A diagrammatic representation of inv(3)(q21;q26); this is an example of a paracentric inversion. Modified from reference 4.

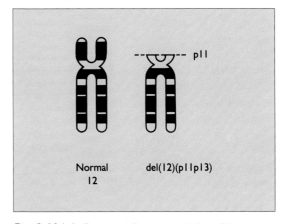

Fig. 3.16 A diagrammatic representation of the del(12)(p11) abnormality. Modified from reference 4.

IMMUNOLOGICAL MARKERS AND FAB CATEGORIES OF MDS

Immunological markers have only a limited place in the diagnosis of MDS and little relationship to the FAB categories. Their only important roles are in identifying circulating micromegakaryocytes and in demonstrating or confirming the nature of blasts, particularly when megakaryoblasts are present or in the uncommon cases in which there is a lymphoblastic or biphenotypic/ bilineage transformation of MDS.

CYTOGENETIC ABNORMALITIES AND THE FAB CATEGORIES OF MDS

Various cytogenetic abnormalities are characteristic of the MDS, among which the commonest anomalies are 5q−, monosomy 5, 7q−, monosomy 7 and trisomy 8 (Fig. 3.17)[72,73,39]. Some abnormalities are particularly characteristic of secondary MDS (Fig. 3.17). The MDS are commonly associated with loss of chromosomal material, either through monosomy, deletion or un- balanced translocation.

There is no close relationship between specific cyto- genetic abnormalities and FAB categories, although some trends are apparent. The frequency with which cyto- genetic abnormalities are observed increases from 20–30 percent in RA, RARS and CMML, to about 45 percent in RAEB and 60–80 percent in RAEB-t. Single abnorm- alities are most likely to be found in RA, RARS and CMML, whereas RAEB-t shows the highest rate of occur- rence of complex rearrangements (whether this is defined as a minimum of 2, 3 or 4 abnormalities in a karyotype). The commonest abnormalities, −5, 5q−, −7, 7q− and +8, are seen in all FAB categories, but 5q− as a single defect is preferentially associated with RA and to a lesser extent with RARS. Such patients often have the features of the 5q− syndrome (female preponderance, macrocytosis, sometimes thrombocytosis, nonlobulated megakaryocytes and relatively good prognosis). Other abnormalities asso- ciated with RA are +8, 20q−, −7, iso(17q) and 17p−. In some series, rearrangements of chromosome 11 have been associated preferentially with RARS, and rearrange- ments of chromosome 12 with CMML.

Other abnormalities are associated with particular clinical or morphological features but not with specific FAB categories. The −7 abnormality is seen in all FAB categories, but in children is associated with a specific syndrome with features of both myeloproliferation and myelodysplasia; in adults it is commonly associated with pancytopenia, a hypocellular bone marrow, trilineage myelodysplasia and a relatively poor prognosis. The 11q− abnormality has been associated with increased ring sideroblasts whether or not the patient falls into the RARS category. Abnormalities of chromosome 3, bands q21 and q26, are associated with thrombocytosis and with increased and abnormal megakaryocytes; the mega- karyocytes (see page 78) are generally smaller than those of the 5q− syndrome although some patients have megakaryocytes with a large round nucleus similar to those of the 5q− syndrome. The translocations t(1;3)(p36;q21), t(6;9)(p21−22;q34) and perhaps also t(1;7)(p11;p11) are associated with a high probability of transformation to AML. Rearrangement of 11q23 is associated specifically with evolution to AML of M4 and M5 categories.

AUTOMATED CYTOCHEMICAL COUNTERS AND FAB CATEGORIES OF ACUTE LEUKAEMIA AND MYELODYSPLASIA

A number of automated cytochemical counters have shown some ability to distinguish between different types of acute leukaemia. The Technicon H.1 counter distin- guishes between different categories of white cell follow- ing a cytochemical reaction for peroxidase. Cells flowing through a narrow beam of light are divided into clusters on the basis of forward light scatter, determined by cell size, and light absorption, determined largely by the intensity of any peroxidase reaction. The positions of clusters of normal cells are shown in Fig. 3.18. Basophils are differentiated from other leucocytes in a separate channel on the basis of the resistance of their cytoplasm to a lytic agent. This channel also assesses the light scatter caused by the stripped nucleus of other leuco- cytes and allows blasts which have hypodense nuclei to be distinguished from other mononuclear cells. Blasts are not counted by the instrument but their suspected presence is 'flagged'. The blast 'flag' is very sensitive to the presence of blast cells but occasionally there is a failure to flag the presence of L1 blasts; very rarely there is a failure to flag the presence of myeloblasts. In some cases the scattergrams may be abnormal despite the failure to flag.

In normal blood very few cells fall into the large unstained cells (LUC) cluster in the peroxidase channel. In ALL (Fig. 3.19), blasts form a spindle or cigar-shaped cluster extending from the lymphocyte area into the LUC area. In the case of L1 ALL many of the blasts are small enough to fall in the lymphocyte area, whereas in L2 ALL a larger proportion are in the LUC area. In L3 the blasts form a more discrete cluster in the LUC area. In AML some blasts lack peroxidase activity and fall into the LUC area while others, depending on the strength of their peroxidase reaction, appear in the monocyte and neutrophil areas (Fig. 3.20). Some leukaemic cells are large so that they appear above the positions of the normal monocyte and neutrophil clusters and others have very intense peroxidase activity so that they fall to the right of the normal neutrophil cluster. Such intense peroxidase activity may be seen in M2 AML and is characteristic of M3. In these cases the mean peroxidase index (MPXI) is elevated. The hypogranular variant of

CYTOGENETIC ABNORMALITIES ASSOCIATED WITH MYELODYSPLASIA			
	Loss of chromosomal material	**Gain of chromosomal material**	**Chromosomal rearrangement**
Common	−5, 5q−* −7, 7q−* 9q− 20q−	+8	
Less common	−Y 1p− 11q− 12p−* 13q− 17p− −20 21q− −22		11q(t) including t(2;11)(p21;q23) and t(11;21)(q24;q11.2) 12p11p13(t)* i(17q) 21q22(t)*

Uncommon or rare	3p−*
	 6p−*
	 −8
	 −14, 14q−
	 −15
	 16q−
	 −17, 17p−, 17q−*
	 18q−
	 −19
	 −21
		Xq13(dup)*
		 +11
		 +16
		 +21
			Xp11(t)*
			 Xq13(t)*
			 der(Y)t(Y;1)(q12;q23)
			 der(1)t(1;7)(p11;p11)*
			 t(1;15)(q12;p11)
			 3p(t)*
			 3q21 or 26 rearrangements including t(1;3)(p36;q21),
			    del(3)(q21), ins(3;3)(q26;q21q26), t(3;4)(q26;q21)
			    and t(3;8)(q26;q24)
			 der(5)t(5;7)(q11.2;p11.2)*
			 6p(t)* including t(6;9)(p23;q34.3)
			 t(11;21)(q24;q11.2)
			 17p(t), 17q(t)*
			 19p(t), 19q(t)*
			 i(21q)
			 ring chromosomes*
			 double minute chromosomes*

*Commoner among cases of secondary MDS. Derived from references 39, 72, 73 and other sources.

Fig. 3.17 Cytogenetic abnormalities associated with myelodysplasia; those which are commoner in secondary myelodysplasia are indicated*.

M3 shows a similar intense peroxidase activity (Fig. 3.21) so that the automated counter provides a rapid means of confirming the diagnosis. Interestingly, M3 and M3V promyelocytes are detected in the basophil/blast channel in the same position as blast cells. M3/M3V are an exception to the general observation that LUC are increased in cases of acute leukaemia, since in these subtypes virtually all leukaemic cells have strong peroxidase activity. The peroxidase channel scattergrams of M4 (Fig. 3.22) and

M5 AML cannot be readily distinguished from those of M1 and M2 although there is a tendency, particularly in M5a AML, for there to be a cluster of very large leukaemic blasts with weak peroxidase activity falling in or on the edge of the LUC area. An eosinophilic component of AML can be readily detected from the peroxidase scattergram (Fig. 3.22). Whether any cases of M0 AML can be distinguished from ALL on the basis of the H.1 peroxidase scattergram has not been established.

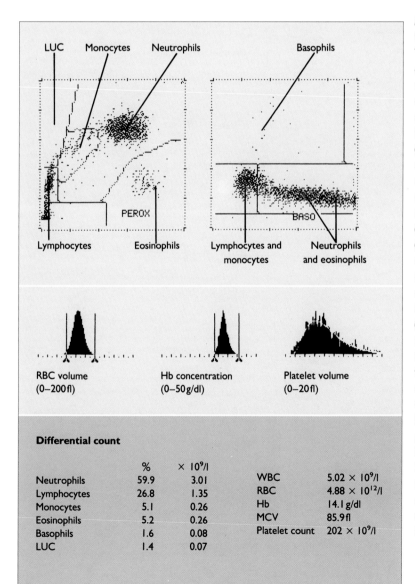

Differential count

	%	× 10⁹/l
Neutrophils	59.9	3.01
Lymphocytes	26.8	1.35
Monocytes	5.1	0.26
Eosinophils	5.2	0.26
Basophils	1.6	0.08
LUC	1.4	0.07

WBC	5.02 × 10⁹/l
RBC	4.88 × 10¹²/l
Hb	14.1 g/dl
MCV	85.9 fl
Platelet count	202 × 10⁹/l

Fig. 3.18 Scattergrams and histograms produced by a Technicon H.1 automated blood-cell counter with a sample of normal blood. In the peroxidase channel (PEROX) forward light scatter (proportional to cell size) is plotted against light absorption (proportional to peroxidase activity). Clusters of cells represent neutrophils, eosinophils, monocytes, lymphocytes and large unstained (i.e. peroxidase-negative) cells (LUC). In the basophil/lobularity channel (BASO) forward light scatter (proportional to size of cell residue) is plotted against high-angle light scatter (proportional to increasing nuclear density/lobulation). Basophils fall above the horizontal threshold. Histograms (lower centre) represent the distribution of red-cell size, red-cell haemoglobin concentration and platelet size. LI is the lobularity index derived in the basophil/lobularity channel. MPXI is a measure of the mean enzymic activity of cells in the peroxidase channel. The LI was 2.71 and the MPXI −1.8.

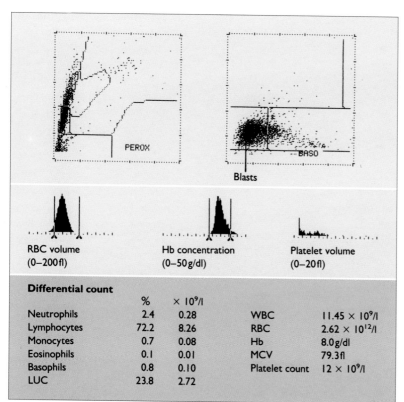

Differential count

	%	× 10⁹/l		
Neutrophils	2.4	0.28	WBC	11.45 × 10⁹/l
Lymphocytes	72.2	8.26	RBC	2.62 × 10¹²/l
Monocytes	0.7	0.08	Hb	8.0 g/dl
Eosinophils	0.1	0.01	MCV	79.3 fl
Basophils	0.8	0.10	Platelet count	12 × 10⁹/l
LUC	23.8	2.72		

Fig. 3.19 Scattergrams and histograms produced by an H.1 automated blood-cell counter with a sample of blood from a patient with L1 ALL. In the peroxidase channel clusters representing neutrophils, eosinophils and monocytes are greatly reduced; blasts fall into the lymphocyte and LUC areas. In the basophil channel cells in the granulocyte area are markedly reduced; blasts fall into the mononuclear cell area and expand the mononuclear cluster to the left generating a blast flag. Severe thrombocytopenia is indicated by the flat histogram of platelet size distribution. The LI was 2.13 and there were flags for microcytes, hyperchromic red cells and blasts. The MPXI was not computed.

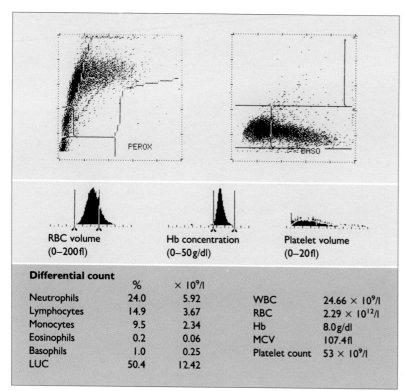

Differential count

	%	× 10⁹/l		
Neutrophils	24.0	5.92	WBC	24.66 × 10⁹/l
Lymphocytes	14.9	3.67	RBC	2.29 × 10¹²/l
Monocytes	9.5	2.34	Hb	8.0 g/dl
Eosinophils	0.2	0.06	MCV	107.4 fl
Basophils	1.0	0.25	Platelet count	53 × 10⁹/l
LUC	50.4	12.42		

Fig. 3.20 Scattergrams and histograms produced by an H.1 automated blood-cell counter with a sample of blood from a patient with M1 AML. In the peroxidase channel some blasts with a low peroxidase content are falling into the LUC area while others with more peroxidase activity appear in the monocyte and neutrophil areas. In the basophil channel blasts have expanded the mononuclear cluster leftwards generating a blast flag. Red cell and platelet histograms show thrombocytopenia and the presence of some macrocytes. Other flags were for anisocytosis, macrocytosis and atypical lymphocytes. LI was 1.33 and MPXI −39.5.

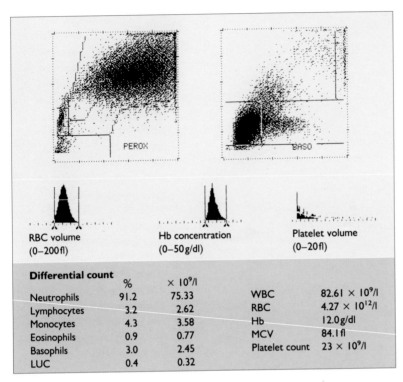

Differential count				
	%	× 10⁹/l		
Neutrophils	91.2	75.33	WBC	82.61 × 10⁹/l
Lymphocytes	3.2	2.62	RBC	4.27 × 10¹²/l
Monocytes	4.3	3.58	Hb	12.0 g/dl
Eosinophils	0.9	0.77	MCV	84.1 fl
Basophils	3.0	2.45	Platelet count	23 × 10⁹/l
LUC	0.4	0.32		

Fig. 3.21 Scattergrams and histograms produced by an H.1 automated blood-cell counter with a sample of blood from a patient with M3V AML. Although the cells were largely agranular they exhibit strong peroxidase activity and form a dense cloud in the neutrophil area extending to the extreme right. In the basophil channels the abnormal promyelocytes appear in the mononuclear area in the same position as blasts and generate a blast flag. They also spill into the basophil area, a phenomenon which may also be seen with blasts. Other flags were for left shift and immature granulocytes. The LI was 1.33 and the MPXI was 10.5.

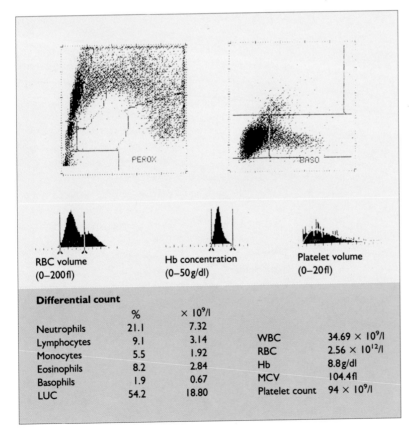

Differential count				
	%	× 10⁹/l		
Neutrophils	21.1	7.32		
Lymphocytes	9.1	3.14	WBC	34.69 × 10⁹/l
Monocytes	5.5	1.92	RBC	2.56 × 10¹²/l
Eosinophils	8.2	2.84	Hb	8.8 g/dl
Basophils	1.9	0.67	MCV	104.4 fl
LUC	54.2	18.80	Platelet count	94 × 10⁹/l

Fig. 3.22 Scattergrams and histograms produced by an H.1 automated blood-cell counter with a sample of blood from a patient with M4Eo AML. In the peroxidase channel, blasts fall into the LUC, monocyte and neutrophil areas; a prominent eosinophil cloud is present which does not separate clearly from the blasts with high peroxidase content. In the basophil channel the blast cloud is not only expanding the mononuclear cluster leftwards but is also stretching upwards to cause a factitious basophilia. The patient was macrocytic and had been transfused hence the dimorphic pattern seen in the histogram of red cell size distribution. There were flags for anisocytosis, macrocytosis, left shift, atypical lymphocytes, blasts and immature granulocytes. The LI was 1.33 and the MPXI −13.2.

In the basophil channel, blasts not only fall to the left of normal mononuclear cells but commonly scatter upwards into the basophil box leading to a factitious elevation of the 'basophil' count (Fig. 3.22). For this reason the automated basophil count in AML is unreliable.

The H.1 counter also permits the detection abnormalities in the MDS (Figs. 3.23 and 3.24). Neutrophils in MDS sometimes have reduced peroxidase activity, leading to a neutrophil cluster which is further to the left than normal and to a reduction in the MPXI, but an elevation of the MPXI has also been described. The presence of blasts in RAEB and RAEB-t may lead to an increase of LUC, a blast 'flag' or, usually, both. The red-cell histograms and scattergrams may show the presence of macrocytosis or a bimodal distribution of cell size or cell haemoglobin concentration which corresponds to the dimorphic blood film associated with sideroblastic erythropoiesis, or there may be increased heterogeneity of red-cell size and haemoglobinization, shown in an increased RDW (red-cell distribution width) and HDW (haemoglobin distribution width), respectively. The platelet histogram may show the presence of giant platelets.

Other automated instruments based on sizing of cells by electrical conductivity or light scatter give similar but not identical information about abnormalities of red cell and platelet size distribution, but give more limited information about white cell characteristics.

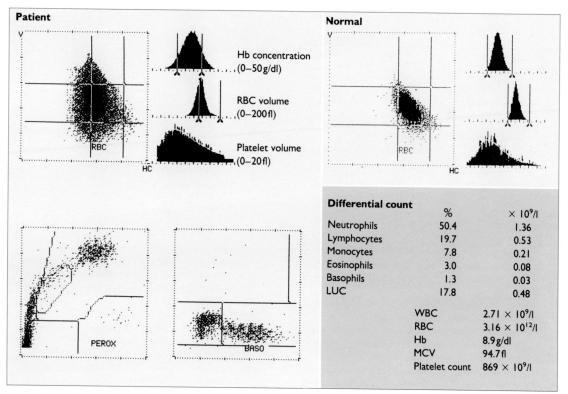

Differential count	%	× 10⁹/l
Neutrophils	50.4	1.36
Lymphocytes	19.7	0.53
Monocytes	7.8	0.21
Eosinophils	3.0	0.08
Basophils	1.3	0.03
LUC	17.8	0.48

WBC	2.71 × 10⁹/l	
RBC	3.16 × 10¹²/l	
Hb	8.9 g/dl	
MCV	94.7 fl	
Platelet count	869 × 10⁹/l	

Fig. 3.23 Scattergrams and histograms produced by an H.1 automated blood-cell counter with a sample of blood from a patient with refractory anaemia; red cell histograms and a red cell scattergram of a normal subject are provided for comparison. In the red cell scattergram, red cell volume (V) is plotted against red cell haemoglobin concentration (HC). The patient has normochromic and hypochromic macrocytes, normochromic and hypo–chromic microcytes and hypochromic cells of normal size. She also shows anaemia, neutropenia and thrombocytosis. There were flags for anisocytosis, microcytosis, macro cytosis and hypochromia. The LI was 2.5 and the MPXI was not computed.

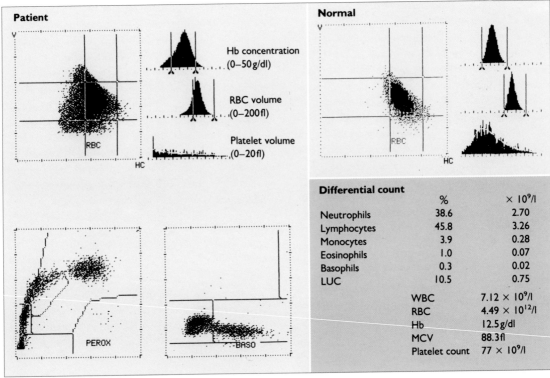

Differential count		
	%	$\times 10^9/l$
Neutrophils	38.6	2.70
Lymphocytes	45.8	3.26
Monocytes	3.9	0.28
Eosinophils	1.0	0.07
Basophils	0.3	0.02
LUC	10.5	0.75
WBC	$7.12 \times 10^9/l$	
RBC	$4.49 \times 10^{12}/l$	
Hb	12.5 g/dl	
MCV	88.3 fl	
Platelet count	$77 \times 10^9/l$	

Fig. 3.24 Scattergrams and histograms produced by an H.I automated blood-cell counter with a sample of blood from a patient with refractory anaemia with ring sideroblasts. The red cell histograms and scattergram show both macrocytes and hypochromic microcytes. The platelet count is severely reduced. There were flags for anisocytosis, microcytosis, macrocytosis and hypochromia. The LI was 2.08 and the MPXI −3.5.

REFERENCES

1. Kristensen JS, Ellegaard J, Hansen KB, Clausen N & Hokland P (1988) First-line diagnosis based on immunological phenotyping in suspected acute leukemia: a prospective study. *Leukemia Research*, **12**, 773–782.

2. Neame PB, Soamboonsrup P, Browman GP, Meyer RM, Benger A, Wilson WEDC, Walker IR, Saeed N & McBride JA (1986) Classifying acute leukemia by immunophenotyping; a combined FAB-immunologic classification of AML. *Blood*, **68**, 1355–1362.

3. First MIC Cooperative Study Group (1986) Morphologic, immunologic, and cytogenetic (MIC) working classification of acute lymphoblastic leukaemias. *Cancer Genetics and Cytogenetics*, **23**, 189–197.

4. Second MIC Cooperative Study Group (1988) Morphologic, immunologic and cytogenetic (MIC) working classification of the acute myeloid leukaemias. *British Journal of Haematology*, **68**, 487–494.

5. Janossy G, Coustan-Smith E & Campana D (1989) The reliability of cytoplasmic CD3 and CD22 antigen expression in the immunodiagnosis of acute leukemia: a study of 500 cases. *Leukemia*, **3**, 170–181.

6. del Vecchio L, Schiavone EM, Ferrara F, Pace E, Lo Pardo C, Pacetti M, Russo M, Cirillo D & Vacca C (1989) Immunodiagnosis of acute leukemia displaying ectopic antigens: proposal for a classification of promiscuous phenotypes. *American Journal of Hematology*, **31**, 173–180.

7. Thiel E, Kranz BR, Raghavachar A, Bartram CR, Löffler H, Messerer D, Ganser A, Ludwig W-D, Büchner T & Hoelzer D (1989) Prethymic phenotype and genotype of pre-T(CD7+/ER−)-cell leukemia and its clinical significance within adult acute lymphoblastic leukemia. *Blood*, **73**, 1247–1258.

8. Pui C-H, Williams DL, Roberson PK, Raimondi SC, Behm FG, Lewis SH, Rivera GK, Kalwinsky DK, Abramowitch M, Crist WM & Murphy SB (1988) Correlation of karyotype and immunotype in childhood acute lymphoblastic leukemia. *Journal of Clinical Oncology*, **6**, 56–61.

9. Carroll AJ, Raimondi SC, Williams DL, Behm FG, Borowitz M, Castleberry RP, Harris MB, Patterson RB, Pullen J & Crist WM (1987) t dic(9;12): a nonrandom chromosome abnormality in childhood B-cell precursor acute lymphoblastic leukemia: a pediatric oncology group study. *Blood*, **70**, 1962–1965.

10. Crist W, Boyett J, Roper M, Pullen J, Metzgar R, Van Eys J, Ragab A, Starling K, Vietti T & Cooper M (1984) Pre-B cell leukemia responds poorly to treatment: a Pediatric Oncology Group study. *Blood*, **63**, 407–414.

11. Crist WM, Shuster JJ, Falletta J, Pullen DJ, Berard CW, Vietti TJ, Alvarado CS, Roper MA, Prasthofer E & Grossi CE (1988) Clinical features and outcome in childhood T-cell leukemia–lymphoma according to the stage of thymocyte differentiation: a pediatric oncology group study. *Blood*, **72**, 1891–1897.

12. Imamura N & Kuramoto A (1988) Acute unclassifiable leukaemia in adults, demonstrating myeloid antigens and myeloperoxidase proteins. *British Journal of Haematology*, **69**, 427–428.

13. Pombo de Oliveira M, Matutes E, Rani S, Morilla R & Catovsky D (1988) Early expression of MCS2 (CD13) in the cytoplasm of blast cells from acute myeloid leukaemia. *Acta Haematologica*, **80**, 61–64.

14. Kemnitz J, Freund M, Helmke Y & Dominis M (1987) Annotations concerning the correlation of the immunophenotypes of leukaemic cells in acute myeloid leukaemias with the FAB classification. *British Journal of Haematology*, **6**, 279.

15. Linch DC, Allen C, Beverley PCL, Bynoe AG, Scott CS & Hogg N (1983) Monoclonal antibodies differentiating between monocytic and myelomonocytic variants of AML. *Blood*, **63**, 566–573.

16. Matutes E, Rodriguez B, Polli N, Tavares de Castro J, Parreira A, Andrews C, Griffin JD, Tindle RW & Catovsky D (1985) Characterization of myeloid leukemias with monoclonal antibodies 3C5 and My9. *Haematological Oncology*, **3**, 179–186.

17. San Miguel JF, Gonzalez M, Canizo MC, Anta JP, Zola H & Lopez Borrasca A (1986) Surface marker analysis in acute myeloid leukaemia and correlation with the FAB classification. *British Journal of Haematology*, **64**, 547–560.

18. Griffin JD, Davis R, Nelson DA, Davey FR, Mayer RJ, Schiffer C, McIntyre OR & Bloomfield CD (1986) Use of surface marker analysis to predict outcome of adult acute myeloblastic leukemia. *Blood*, **68**, 1232–1241.

19. Vainchenker W, Villeval JL, Tabilio A, Matamis H, Karianakis G, Guichard J, Henri A, Vernant JP, Rochant H & Breton-Gorius J (1988) Immunophenotype of leukemic blast cells with small peroxidase-positive granules detected by electron microscopy. *Leukemia*, **2**, 274–281.

20. Campos L. Guyotat D, Archimbaud E, Devaux Y, Treille D, Larise A, Maupas J, Gentilhomme O, Ehrsam A & Fiere D (1989) Surface marker expression in adult acute myeloid leukaemia: correlations with initial characteristics, morphology and response to therapy. *British Journal of Haematology*, **72**, 161–166.

21. Krause JR, Stolc V, Kaplan SS & Penchansky L (1989) Microgranular promyelocytic leukemia: a multiparameter examination. *American Journal of Hematology*, **30**, 158–163.

22. Erber WN, Breton-Gorius J, Villeval JL, Oscier DG, Bai Y & Mason DY (1987) Detection of cells of megakaryocyte lineage in haematological malignancies by immuno-alkaline phosphatase labelling cell smears with a panel of monoclonal antibodies. *British Journal of Haematology*, **65**, 87–94.

23. Villeval JL, Testa U, Vinci G, Tonthat H, Bettaieb A, Titeux M, Cramer P, Edelman L, Rochant H, Breton-Gorius J & Vainchenker W (1985) Carbonic anhydrase I is an early marker of normal human erythroid differentiation. *Blood*, **66**, 1162–1170.

24. Imamura N, Inada T, Mtasiwa DM & Kuramoto A (1989) Demonstration of thrombospondin (TSP) receptor on the cell surface of acute megakaryoblastic leukemia. *American Journal of Hematology*, **31**, 142–143.

25. Das Gupta A, Samoszuk MK, Papayannopoulou T & Stamatoyannopoulos G (1985) SFL23.6: a monoclonal antibody reactive with CFU-E, erythroblasts and erythrocytes. *Blood*, **66**, 522–526.

26. Mirro J & Kitchingman GR (1989) The morphology, cytochemistry, molecular characteristics and clinical significance of acute mixed-lineage leukaemia. In *Leukaemia Cytochemistry: Principles and Practice*, edited by CS Scott. Ellis Horwood Limited, Chichester.

27. Berger R, Bernheim A, Daniel M-T, Valensi F & Flandrin G (1981) Karyotype and cell phenotypes in primary acute leukemias. *Blood Cells*, **7**, 287–292.

28. Bitter MA, Le Beau MM, Rowley JD, Larson RA, Golomb HM & Vardiman JW (1987) Associations between morphology, karyotype, and clinical features in myeloid leukemias. *Human Pathology*, **18**, 211–225.

29. Standing Committee on Human Cytogenetic Nomenclature (1978) An international system for human cytogenetic nomenclature. *Cytogenetics and Cell Genetics*, **21**, 309–404.

30. Raimondi SC, Behm FG, Roberson PK, Pui C-H, Rivera GK, Murphy SB & Williams DL (1988) Cytogenetics of childhood T-cell leukemia. *Blood*, **72**, 1560–1566.

31. Uckun FM, Gajl-Peczalska J, Provisor AJ & Heerema NA (1988) Immunophenotype-karyotype association in human acute lymphoblastic leukemia. *Blood*, **73**, 271–280.

32. Kocova M. Kowalczyk JR & Sandberg AA (1985) Translocation 4;11 acute leukemia: three case reports and review of the literature. *Cancer Genetics and Cytogenetics*, **16**, 21–32.

33. Katz F, Malcolm S, Gibbons B, Tilly R, Lam G, Robertson ME, Czepulkowski B & Chessels J (1988) Cellular and molecular studies on infant null acute lymphoblastic leukaemia. *Blood*, **71**, 1438–1447.

34. Umiel T, Nadler LM, Cohen IJ, Levine H, Stark B, Mammon Z, Dzaldetti M, Rechavi G, Simone F, Katzir N, Ramot B & Zaizov R (1987) Undifferentiated leukemia of infancy with t(11;17) chromosomal rearrangement coexpressing myeloid and B restricted antigens. *Cancer*, **59**, 1143–1149.

35. Bloomfield CD et al. (1986) Chromosome abnormalities identify high-risk and low-risk patients with acute lymphoblastic leukemia. *Blood*, **67**, 415–420.

36. Fenaux P, Lai JL, Morel P, Nelken B, Taboureau O, Deminatti M & Bauters F (1989) Cytogenetics and their prognostic value in childhood and adult acute lymphoblastic leukemia (ALL) excluding L3. *Hematological Oncology*, **7**, 307–317.

37. Secker-Walker LM, Chessels JM, Stewart EL, Swansbury GJ, Richards S & Lawler SD (1989) Chromosomes and other prognostic features in acute lymphoblastic leukaemia; a long-term follow-up. *British Journal of Haematology*, **72**, 336–342.

38. Williams DL, Harber J, Murphy SB, Look T, Kalwinsky DK, Rivera G, Melvin SL, Stass S & Dahl GV (1986) Chromosomal translocations play a unique role in influencing prognosis in childhood acute lymphoblastic leukemia. *Blood*, **68**, 205–212.

39. Yunis JJ, Lobell M, Arnesen MA, Oken MM, Mayer MG, Rydell RE & Brunning RD (1988) Refined chromosome study helps define prognostic subgroups in most patients with primary myelodysplastic syndrome and acute myelogenous leukaemia. *British Journal of Haematology*, **68**, 189–194.

40. Fourth International Workshop on Chromosomes in Leukemia, 1982 (1984) Clinical significance of chromosome abnormalities in acute nonlymphocytic leukemia. *Cancer Genetics and Cytogenetics*, **11**, 332–350.

41. Schiffer CA, Lee EJ, Tomiyasu T, Wiernik PH & Testa JR (1989) Prognostic impact of cytogenetic abnormalities in patients with de novo acute nonlymphocytic leukemia. Blood, **73**, 263–270.

42. Fenaux P, Preudhomme CV, Lai JL, Morel P, Beuscart R & Bauters F (1989) Cytogenetics and their prognostic value in de novo acute myeloid leukaemia: a report on 283 cases. British Journal of Haematology, **73**, 61–67.

43. Trujillo JM, Cork A, Ahearn MJ, Youness EL, McCredia KB (1979) Hematologic and cytologic characterization of 8/21 translocation acute granulocytic leukemia. Blood, **53**, 695–706.

44. Berger R, Bernheim A, Daniel M-T, Valensi F, Sigaux F & Flandrin G (1982) Cytological characterization and significance of normal karyotypes in t(8;21) acute myeloblastic leukaemia. Blood, **59**, 171–178.

45. Fourth International Workshop on Chromosomes in Leukemia, 1982 (1984) Translocation (8;21)(q22;q22) in acute nonlymphocytic leukemia. Cancer Genetics and Cytogenetics, **11**, 284–287.

46. Swirsky DM, Li YS, Matthews JG, Flemans RJ, Rees JHK & Hayhoe FGJ (1984) 8;21 translocation in acute granulocytic leukaemia: cytological, cytochemical and clinical features. British Journal of Haematology, **56**, 199–213.

47. Berger R, Flandrin G, Bernheim A, Le Coniat M, Vecchione D, Pacot A, Derré J, Daniel M-T, Valensi F, Sigaux F & Ochoa-Noguera ME (1987) Cytogenetic studies on 519 consecutive de novo acute nonlymphocytic leukemias. Cancer Genetics and Cytogenetics, **29**, 9–21.

48. Li Y-S & Yang C-L (1987) Consistent chromosomal changes in Chinese patients with acute nonlymphocytic leukemia. Cancer Genetics and Cytogenetics, **26**, 379–380.

49. Kaneko Y, Kimpara H, Kawai S & Fujimoto T (1983) 8;21 chromosome translocation in eosinophilic leukemia. Cancer Genetics and Cytogenetics, **9**, 181–183.

50. Jacobsen RJ, Temple MJ & Sacher RA (1984) Acute myeloblastic leukaemia and t(8;21) translocation. British Journal of Haematology, **57**, 539–540.

51. Hayhoe FGJ & Quaglino D (1988) Haematological Cytochemistry, Second Edition. Churchill Livingstone, Edinburgh.

52. Kamada N, Dohy H, Okada K, Oguma N, Kuramoto A, Tanaku K & Uchino H (1981) In vivo and in vitro activity of neutrophil alkaline phosphatase in acute myelocytic leukemia with 8;21 translocation. Blood, **58**, 1213–1217.

53. Berger R, Bernheim A, Sigaux F, Daniel M-T, Valensi F & Flandrin G (1982) Acute monocytic leukemia; chromosome studies. Leukemia Research, **6**, 17–26.

54. Le Beau MM, Larson RA, Bitter MA, Vardiman JW, Golomb HM & Rowley JD (1983) Association of an inversion of chromosome 16 with abnormal marrow eosinophils in acute myelomonocytic leukemia. New England Journal of Medicine, **309**, 630–636.

55. Arthur DC & Bloomfield CD (1983) Partial deletion of the long arm of chromosome 16 and bone marrow eosinophilia in acute nonlymphocytic leukemia: a new association. Blood, **61**, 994–998.

56. Matsuura Y, Sato N, Kimura F, Shimomura S, Yamamoto K, Enomoto Y & Takatani O (1987) An increase in basophils in a case of acute myelomonocytic leukaemia associated with bone marrow eosinophilia and inversion of chromosome 16. European Journal of Haematology, **39**, 457–461.

57. Ohyashiki K, Ohyashiki JH, Kondo M, Ito H & Toyama K (1988) Chromosome change at 16q22 in nonlymphocytic leukemia: clinical implications on leukemia patients with inv(16) versus del(16). Leukemia, **2**, 35–40.

58. Sandberg AA, Hecht B KMc-C & Hecht F (1985) Nomenclature: the Philadelphia chromosome or Ph without superscript. Cancer Genetics and Cytogenetics, **14**, 1.

59. Sasaki M, Kondo K & Tomiyasu T (1983) Cytogenetic characterization of 10 cases of Ph¹-positive acute myelogenous leukemia. Cancer Genetics and Cytogenetics, **9**, 119–128.

60. Pearson MG, Vardiman JW, Le Beau MM, Rowley JD, Schwartz S, Kerman SL, Cohen MM, Fleischman EW & Prigogina EL (1985) Increased numbers of marrow basophils may be associated with a t(6;9) in ANLL. American Journal of Hematology, **18**, 393–403.

61. Heim S, Kristoffersson U, Mandahl N, Mitelman F, Bekassy AN, Garwicz S & Wiebe T (1986) High resolution banding analysis of the reciprocal translocation t(6;9) in acute nonlymphocytic leukemia. Cancer Genetics and Cytogenetics, **22**, 195–201.

62. Horsman DE & Kalousek DK (1987) Acute myelomonocytic leukemia (AML-M4) and translocation t(6;9)(p23;q34): two additional patients with prominent myelodysplasia. Cancer Genetics and Cytogenetics, **26**, 77–82.

63. Jenkins RB, Tefferi A, Solberg LA & Dewald GW (1989) Acute leukemia with abnormal thrombopoiesis and inversions of chromosome 3. Cancer Genetics and Cytogenetics, **39**, 167–179.

64. Bloomfield CD, Garson DM, Volin L, Knuutila S, de la Chapelle A (1985) t(1;3)(p36;q21) in acute nonlymphocytic leukemia: a new cytogenetic-clinicopathologic association. Blood, **66**, 1409–1413.

65. Hoyle CF, Sherrington P & Hayhoe FGJ (1988) Translocation (3;6)(q21;p21) in acute myeloid leukemia with abnormal thrombopoiesis and basophilia. Cancer Genetics and Cytogenetics, **30**, 261–267.

66. Hoyle C, Sherrington PD & Hayhoe FGJ (1987) Cytological features of 9q– deletions in AML. Blood, **60**, 277–278.

67. Sato Y, Abe S, Mise K, Sasaki M, Kamada N, Kouda K, Musashi M, Saburi Y, Horikoshi A, Minami Y, Miyakuni T, Yokoyama Y, Ishihara I & Miura Y (1987) Reciprocal translocation involving the short arms of chromosomes 7 and 11, t(7p–;11p+) associated with myeloid leukemia with maturation. Blood, **70**, 1654–1658.

68. Raimondi SC, Dubé ID, Valentine MD, Mirro J, Watt HJ, Larson RA, Bitter MA, Le Beau MM & Rowley JD (1989) Clinicopathologic manifestations of the t(3;5) in patients with acute nonlymphocytic leukemia. Leukemia, **3**, 42–47.

69. Archimbaud E, Charrin C, Guyotat D, Magaud J-P, Gentilhomme O & Fiere D (1988) Acute leukaemia with t(4;11) in patients previously exposed to carcinogens. British Journal of Haematology, **69**, 467–470.

70. Bastard G, Vannier JP, Bizet M, Lenorman B & Tron P (1985) Translocation (4;11;17) in a case of acute lymphoblastic leukemia. Cancer Genetics and Cytogenetics, **1**, 81–82.

71. Daeschner C, Elder F, Carpenteri U & Haggard ME (1985) Leukemia with a novel 4q11q rearrangement. Cancer Genetics and Cytogenetics, **16**, 245–250.

72. Musilova J & Michalova K (1988) Chromosome study of 85 patients with myelodysplastic syndromes. Cancer Genetics and Cytogenetics, **33**, 39–50.

73. Third MIC Cooperative Study Group (1988) Recommendations for a morphologic, immunologic and cytogenetic (MIC) working classification of the primary and therapy-related myelodysplastic disorders. Cancer Genetics and Cytogenetics, **32**, 1–10.

chapter four

CHRONIC LYMPHOID

LEUKAEMIAS

In 1989 the FAB group published proposals for the classification of chronic B and T lymphoid leukaemias[1]. The classification is based on clinical features, cell morphology, membrane markers and histology. Some of the categories identified are associated with specific cytogenetic abnormalities. The chronic lymphoid leukaemias are broadly separated into B lineage and T lineage.

CHRONIC LEUKAEMIAS OF B-LYMPHOCYTE LINEAGE

Chronic leukaemias of B-lymphocyte lineage usually express membrane immunoglobulin and occasionally cytoplasmic immunoglobulin. They also express a variety of antigenic markers recognized by monoclonal antibodies (McAb), some of which are shared with T lymphocytes or with other haemopoietic cells, and some of which are specific for B-lineage cells. A further cell-membrane marker not yet identifiable by means of McAb can be recognized by a rosetting technique with mouse red blood cells. Some of the immunological markers used for characterizing leukaemic and normal lymphocytes give positive reactions with B lymphocytes and their precursors, some are positive only with mature B cells, and some show selectivity for subsets of normal B lymphocytes and for specific categories of lymphoproliferative disorder (Fig. 4.1). The expression of immunoglobulin (Ig) in leukaemic cells is monoclonal, that is it is restricted to a single light chain type ($\varkappa$ or λ) although there may be more than one type of heavy chain (μ, δ, α, γ). DNA analysis shows that in chronic lymphoid leukaemia of B lineage the Ig heavy chain and usually the light chain genes have undergone rearrangement; in some cases the

gene for the β chain of the T-cell receptor has also been rearranged.

The chronic leukaemias of B lineage can be further categorized on the basis of clinical features, cell morphology, cell markers and histology. Characteristic immunological markers in each category are summarized in Fig. 4.2. Leukaemias of mature B cells are negative for terminal deoxynucleotidyl transferase (TdT) which is characteristically positive in acute lymphoblastic leukaemia.

Chronic lymphocytic leukaemia

Chronic lymphocytic leukaemia (CLL) is by far the commonest of the chronic B-cell leukaemias. It is typically a disease of the elderly which, in its later stages, is characterized by lymphadenopathy, hepatomegaly and splenomegaly and eventual impairment of bone marrow function. Various arbitrary levels of absolute lymphocyte count have been suggested for the diagnosis of CLL (for example $>10 \times 10^9/l$), but the demonstration of a monoclonal population of B lymphocytes with characteristic markers allows the disease to be diagnosed at an earlier stage when the lymphocyte count is less elevated.

MORPHOLOGY

In CLL the leukaemic cells are typically small with a conspicuous, though usually narrow, rim of cytoplasm[1] (Fig. 4.3). The cell morphology is more uniform than that of normal peripheral blood lymphocytes. The nuclear and cytoplasmic outlines are generally regular although

SOME MONOCLONAL ANTIBODIES USED IN THE CHARACTERIZATION OF CHRONIC LYMPHOID LEUKAEMIAS OF B LINEAGE

Cluster designation	Representative McAb	Specificity within haemopoietic lineage
CD19, CD20, CD24	see Fig. 3.1	B lineage (see Fig. 3.1) (granulocytes are also reactive with CD24)
unclustered†	HLA-Dr, OKIa, GRB1, FMC4	anti-HLA-Dr (Ia): virtually all B lymphocytes and their precursors, plasma cells, activated T cells, haemopoietic precursors, monocytes
unclustered	anti-Ig*, anti-γ, α, μ, δ, κ, λ*	immunoglobulin and its constituent chains: SmIg is a pan-B marker; cytoplasmic Ig is detectable in pre-B cells (Cy μ) and in plasma cells (CyIg); anti-γ, α, μ, δ, κ, λ identify subsets of B cells and are useful for demonstrating clonality
CD5†	OKT1, OKT101, Leu 1, UCHT2, OKCLL	thymocytes and T lymphocytes, many T-cell malignancies, a small subset of B cells, the majority of cases of B-CLL and intermediate lymphoma, a minority of cases of B-PLL
CD23	Blast-2, PL-13, MHM 6, Tü 1	low affinity $Fc_\varepsilon R$: activated B cells, majority of cases of CLL and CLL-PL, minority of cases of PLL and NHL
CD21	B2, RFB6, BA-5	CR2 (C3dR): subset of B cells, majority of cases of CLL, about 50 percent of cases of NHL
CD22	To15, Leu 14, RFB-4	most mature B cells and some B-cell precursors (see Fig. 3.1), NHL, HCL and B-PLL
CD10	J5, OKB-CALLA, BA-3, VIL-A1, NU-N1	common ALL antigen (CALLA) but also expressed on some NHL, particularly follicular lymphomas and some plasma cell leukaemias and myeloma cells
unclustered	FMC7	small subset of B cells, majority of cases of NHL, HCL and B-PLL
CD25†	anti-Tac, Tac1, IL-2R1	interleukin 2 receptor: activated T and B cells, hairy cells, ATLL cells
CD38†	OKT10	activated T and B cells, plasma cells, haemopoietic precursors, thymic cells

† also positive in some T lymphocytes
* some polyclonal antisera are in current use

ALL, acute lymphoblastic leukaemia; ATLL, adult T-cell leukaemia lymphoma; CLL, chronic lymphocytic leukaemia; PLL, prolymphocytic leukaemia; HCL, hairy cell leukaemia; NHL, non-Hodgkin's lymphoma.

Fig. 4.1   Some monoclonal antibodies used in the characterization of chronic leukaemias of B lineage.

some cases have somewhat indented nuclei. Nuclear chromatin is dense and clumped in coarse blocks, with nucleoli usually inconspicuous or not visible on light microscopy. The cytoplasm is weakly basophilic and sometimes contains small vacuoles. CLL lymphocytes are more fragile than normal lymphocytes and thus the formation of smudge cells or smear cells during the spreading of the blood film is common; this feature is not pathognomonic but can be helpful in diagnosis. The presence of up to 10 percent of prolymphocytes (see below) is compatible with the diagnosis of CLL.

IMMUNOPHENOTYPE OF CHRONIC B-CELL LEUKAEMIAS

Marker	CLL	PLL	HCL	follicular lymphoma	intermediate lymphoma	SLVL	plasma cell leukaemia
SmIg	weak	strong	strong	strong	moderate	strong	negative
CyIg	–	–/+	–/+	–	–	–/+	++
MRFC	++	–	–/+	–/+	–/+	–	–
CD5	++	–/+	–	–	++	–	–
CD19,20,24	++	++	++*	++	++	++	–
HLA-Dr (Ia)	++	++	++	++	++	++	–
FMC7,CD22	–/+	++	++	+	+	++	–
CD10	–	–/+	–	+	–/+	–	–/+
CD25	–	–	++	–	–	–/+	–
CD38	–	–	–/+	–/+	–	–/+	++

The frequency with which a marker is positive in >30 percent of cells in a particular leukaemia is indicated as follows: ++ 80–100 percent; + 40–80 percent; –/+ 10–40 percent; – 0–9 percent.

* It is possible that HCL cells are negative with CD24 McAb since negative reactions are obtained with L30, a McAb which probably belongs to this cluster.

CLL, chronic lymphocytic leukaemia; PLL, prolymphocytic leukaemia; HCL, hairy cell leukaemia; SLVL, splenic lymphoma with villous lymphocytes; MRFC, mouse rosette forming cells.

Fig. 4.2   Characteristic immunological phenotype in chronic leukaemias of B lineage. Derived from Bennett et al[1].

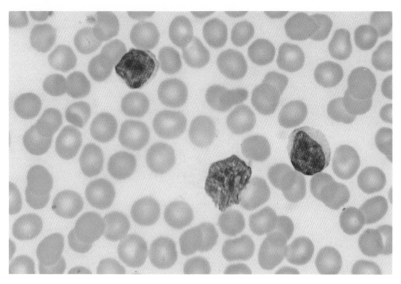

Fig. 4.3   PB film in chronic lymphocytic leukaemia showing two mature lymphocytes and one smear cell. Nuclear chromatin is condensed and each cell contains a barely detectable nucleolus. MGG × 960.

CELL MARKERS

CLL cells[1] (Fig. 4.2) express surface membrane immunoglobulin (SmIg) weakly; the heavy chain most often expressed is μ, with or without δ. The cells are positive with McAb which identify the B lineage such as CD19, CD20 and CD24. In addition the great majority of cases are positive with CD5 (also reactive with T-lineage cells), CD21 and CD23. Reactivity with FMC7 and the pan-B marker CD22 are uncommon. In the great majority of cases cells form rosettes with mouse red blood cells (MRFC).

HISTOLOGY

The bone marrow is hypercellular as a consequence of lymphoid infiltration. The pattern of infiltration is either interstitial, nodular, mixed nodular and interstitial, or diffuse. The term interstitial indicates that leukaemic cells are infiltrating between the normal haemopoietic cells without disturbing the architecture of the bone marrow. Diffuse, on the other hand, is used to designate heavy infiltration which effaces the fat spaces and destroys normal bone marrow architecture; the term 'packed marrow' has also been used to describe this histological appearance. The pattern of infiltration correlates with the stage of the disease, with interstitial or nodular infiltration being seen in the earliest stages of the disease and a packed marrow pattern in the later stages. Lymph node biopsies show diffuse infiltration with obliteration of the normal architecture. The spleen shows a variable infiltration of the red and white pulp; either may predominate[2]. The infiltration in the white pulp may be nodular[3].

CYTOGENETICS

The commonest cytogenetic abnormalities in CLL are trisomy 12 and a variety of translocations which have in common a breakpoint at 14q32, the site of the Ig heavy chain locus; among these t(11;14)(q13;q32) is most common. Other relatively common abnormalities are 6q−, 11q− and rearrangements involving various breakpoints on chromosome 13.

Chronic lymphocytic leukaemia, mixed cell types

In some cases which otherwise appear typical of CLL there is an increase in prolymphocytes so that they constitute more than 10 percent of lymphoid cells (designated CLL/PL)[4,5]; in others there is a spectrum of cells from small to large lymphocytes, with a tendency to cytoplasmic basophilia but with less than 10 percent of cells being prolymphocytes. These two groups of patients have been categorized by the FAB group as CLL, mixed cell type[1]. Cases with more than 55 percent of prolymphocytes fall into the prolymphocytic leukaemia (PLL) category (see below). The prolymphocytes of CLL/

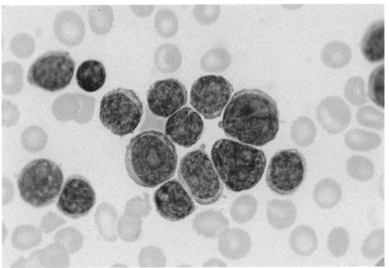

Fig. 4.4 PB film in B-prolymphocytic leukaemia showing cells which are regular in shape with round nuclei. Nuclear chromatin shows some condensation and the larger cells contain prominent vesicular nucleoli. MGG × 960.

PL are more pleomorphic than those of PLL, and the small lymphocytes, when sized by impedance technology, are larger than those of CLL. CLL/PL includes patients who present *de novo* with this morphology and others who undergo a 'prolymphocytoid transformation' of CLL. It is suggested that patients with CLL/PL may have a worse prognosis than patients with typical CLL[1], but a worse prognostic significance has not been recognized for patients who have an admixture of larger lymphocytes.

CELL MARKERS

About two-thirds of cases of CLL/PL have an immunological phenotype which is typical of CLL. The other third show atypical features such as strong expression of SmIg or expression of FMC7. The immunological phenotype in patients who have a spectrum of cell size has not been defined.

Prolymphocytic leukaemia

PLL[6] has a higher median age of onset than CLL. It is characterized by a high white cell count, very specific morphological features and marked splenomegaly with only trivial lymphadenopathy.

MORPHOLOGY

The predominant cell is the prolymphocyte[1] (Fig. 4.4); 55 percent of circulating prolymphocytes was found to be the best figure to distinguish between PLL and CLL/PL[5]. The prolymphocyte is a large cell with cytoplasm which is relatively more abundant than that of a CLL cell. The nucleus is round with a prominent vesicular nucleolus and moderately well condensed nuclear chromatin.

CELL MARKERS

About two-thirds of cases of B-PLL have an immunological phenotype which differs markedly from that of CLL[1] (Fig. 4.2). SmIg is strong, MRFC and CD5 expression are low and FMC7 expression is high. The SmIg is usually μ with or without δ. In the other third of cases the immunological phenotype is intermediate between the typical CLL phenotype and the typical PLL phenotype.

HISTOLOGY

The bone marrow is hypercellular with the most common pattern of infiltration being interstitial/nodular or diffuse; interstitial and interstitial/diffuse patterns are also seen. Reticulin is much more often increased than in CLL. Lymph node infiltration is diffuse with or without a pseudonodular pattern. Splenic infiltration is in both the red and white pulp, with large proliferative nodules in the white pulp showing a characteristic bizonal appearance, dense at the centre and lighter at the periphery consequent on the larger cells being peripheral[2].

CYTOGENETICS

B-PLL shows a high incidence of complex karyotypic abnormalities and of clonal evolution[7]. Trisomy 12 which is common in CLL is much less common in PLL. Translocations involving chromosome 14 with a breakpoint at 14q32 are common but are more often found in a sideline than in the stemline; those which have been observed include t(11;14)(q13;q32), t(12;14)(q22;q32) and t(14;17) (q32;q11). Other relatively common abnormalities have included t/del(12)(p12–13), del(6)(q21) and del(3)(p13).

Hairy cell leukaemia

Hairy cell leukaemia (HCL) occurs throughout adult life. It is characterized by splenomegaly with little lymphadenopathy. Circulating leukaemic cells are not usually numerous and many patients are pancytopenic. Severe monocytopenia is usual.

MORPHOLOGY

Hairy cells are larger than normal lymphocytes or CLL lymphocytes. They have moderately abundant, weakly basophilic cytoplasm with irregular 'hairy' projections and consequently an ill-defined cell outline (Fig. 4.5). The cytoplasm may contain azurophilic granules or weakly basophilic rod-shaped inclusions. The nucleus is eccentric, and round, oval, dumbbell or kidney-shaped. The nuclear chromatin has a finely dispersed pattern and nucleoli are inconspicuous, small and usually single. The bone marrow is usually difficult to aspirate as a consequence of fibrosis, but when it can be aspirated hairy cells are relatively more numerous than in the blood.

CYTOCHEMISTRY

In the great majority of cases of HCL the cells show tartrate-resistant acid phosphatase (TRAP) activity. TRAP activity is also observed in some cases of hairy cell variant, in a proportion of cells in a minority of cases of PLL, and rarely in other lymphoproliferative disorders.

CELL MARKERS

Hairy cells have the immunological phenotype of a relatively mature B cell[1] (Fig. 4.2). SmIg is strongly expressed with some cases also showing cytoplasmic immunoglobulin (CyIg). In about one-third of cases the SmIg heavy chain is μ with or without δ, while the remainder of cases express either γ or α. CD5, CD21 and CD23 are negative. FMC7 and CD22 are positive, as is CD25 (anti-Tac), a marker of activated T and B cells, which is uncommonly positive in other B-cell leukaemias. There are several markers which show a degree of specificity for hairy cells; they include anti-HC2 and LeuM5 (CD11c), both of which are also positive in monocytes. In addition, hairy cells may give positive reactions with several McAb which are also reactive with plasma cells including PCA-1 and BU11.

HISTOLOGY

The bone marrow biopsy shows a highly characteristic pattern of diffuse infiltration with nuclei of cells appearing to be spaced apart and each cell being surrounded by a clear zone (Fig. 4.6). This pattern is more apparent on paraffin-embedded specimens than in plastic-embedded specimens although the latter show the cellular detail more clearly. Reticulin is increased. Occasional patients show only patchy focal infiltration or have a very hypocellular but infiltrated bone marrow. Spleen histology shows a distinctive pattern of red pulp infiltration with widening of the pulp cords and the formation of pseudosinuses lined by hairy cells.

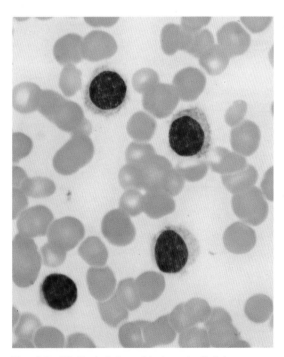

Fig. 4.5 PB film in hairy cell leukaemia. Cells have round nuclei with condensed chromatin and moderately abundant cytoplasm with ragged edges. MGG × 960.

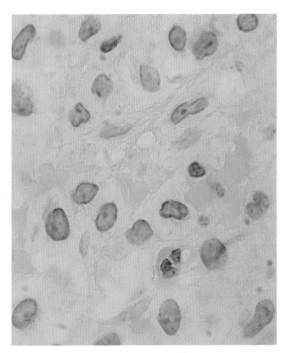

Fig. 4.6 Bone marrow trephine biopsy in hairy cell leukaemia showing cells with round, oval or irregular nuclei surrounded by scanty, ragged cytoplasm. The spacing of the nuclei is characteristic of HCL. Two neutrophils and one erythroblast are also present. Paraffin-embedded, H&E, × 960.

A variety of chromosomal abnormalities have been described in HCL but no consistent association has been recognized. Some cases have had translocations involving a 14q23 breakpoint, but not necessarily in the stemline.

Hairy cell leukaemia variant

Hairy cell variant (HCV)[1,8,9], like HCL, is characterized by splenomegaly with little lymphadenopathy. In contrast to HCL the white cell count is usually high with leukaemic cells being numerous in the peripheral blood, and the monocyte count is usually normal. Evidence is also emerging that both alpha interferon and deoxycoformycin therapy, which are highly successful in HCL, are often ineffective in HCV[1,9]. The latter can be confused not only with HCL but also with splenic lymphoma with villous lymphocytes.

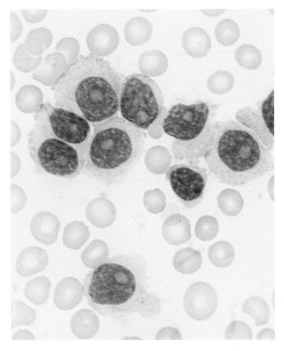

Fig. 4.7 PB film in hairy cell leukaemia variant. Cells are nucleolated and it is evident that the white cell count is high. MGG × 960.

The cells of HCV have a higher nucleocytoplasmic ratio than classical hairy cells, the cytoplasm is more basophilic and the nucleus has a more condensed chromatin pattern with a prominent nucleolus (Fig. 4.7). The nucleus, in fact, shows more resemblance to that of a typical B-PLL prolymphocyte than that of a classical hairy cell. TRAP is usually negative but in some cases is positive.

The immunological phenotype is closer to that of PLL than to that of classical HCL. Negative reactions are usual with CD25 and anti-HC2 although some cases are LeuM5 (CD11c) positive and, in common with classical HCL, reactions with L30 are negative[10]. The majority of cases express γ heavy chain[9].

The pattern of infiltration in the spleen is similar to that of HCL but without the formation of pseudosinuses. The pattern of bone marrow infiltration also differs; infiltrating cells are clumped together with an interstitial or diffuse/nodular pattern[9].

Splenic lymphoma with villous lymphocytes

As suggested by the name, splenic lymphoma with villous lymphocytes (SLVL)[11] is a predominantly splenic lymphoma with lymphadenopathy being minor. The white cell count varies from normal to moderately elevated, with the majority of circulating cells being abnormal lymphocytes. SLVL is commonly confused with B-CLL but has distinctive clinical and pathological features.

Cells are larger than CLL cells. The nucleus is round to ovoid with clumped chromatin and, in about half the cases, a distinct small nucleolus[1] (Fig. 4.8). The cytoplasm varies in amount, is moderately basophilic and has short villous projections often localized at one pole of the cell. The nucleocytoplasmic ratio is higher than in HCL or HCV. A minority of cells show plasmacytoid features, that is the nucleus is eccentric, basophilia is more pronounced and a Golgi zone is apparent. TRAP is negative.

CELL MARKERS

The SLVL cell corresponds to a relatively mature B cell (Fig. 4.2). SmIg is strong, CyIg is sometimes expressed and about two-thirds of cases have a monoclonal Ig in the serum or the urine. Overall, membrane markers are similar to those of prolymphocytes.

HISTOLOGY

In contrast to CLL, the bone marrow is infiltrated in only about one-half of cases. The pattern of infiltration can be either nodular or diffuse. In contrast to CLL, PLL, HCL and HCV, splenic infiltration is often predominantly in the white pulp[1,2]. Plasmacytoid differentiation is often more prominent in histological sections than in peripheral blood cells.

Non-Hodgkin's lymphoma in leukaemic phase

Various types of non-Hodgkin's lymphoma have circulating lymphoma cells at presentation or subsequently enter a leukaemic phase. The likelihood of leukaemic manifestations varies between different types of lymphoma, but is relatively high in those small-cell lymphomas in which the phenotype of the malignant cells corresponds to that of a relatively mature B cell, for example follicular lymphoma (small-cell type) or intermediate lymphoma (mantle-zone lymphoma, diffuse centrocytic lymphoma). A leukaemic phase is considerably less common in large cell lymphomas. The leukaemic phase of Burkitt's lymphoma is excluded from the FAB classification of chronic (mature) B lymphoid leukaemias since it corresponds to the phenotype of acute lymphoblastic leukaemia, L3 subtype. The clinical features of lymphoma in leukaemic phase are determined largely by the nature of the lymphoma. They usually include lymphadenopathy, splenomegaly, or both, although occasional cases are diagnosed from an incidental blood film before any organomegaly has occurred.

MORPHOLOGY

The leukaemic phases of small-cell follicular lymphoma and of intermediate/mantle-zone lymphoma have been well characterized. The circulating cells of follicular lymphoma[12] (Fig. 4.9) are more pleomorphic than CLL cells. They range in size from cells which are distinctly smaller than those of CLL, the nuclei of which are small with uniformly condensed chromatin and very scanty cytoplasm, to larger cells with more abundant cytoplasm. Cells may be either round or angular. Nucleoli are usually not visible. A variable, often large proportion of the cells have nuclei with deep, narrow clefts or fissures. Diagnosis of the leukaemic phase of intermediate or

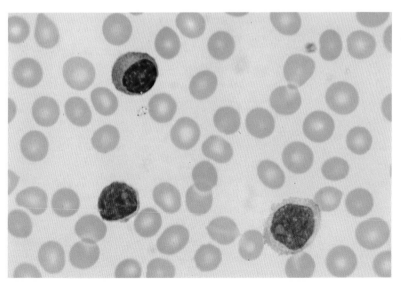

Fig. 4.8 PB film in splenic lymphoma with villous lymphocytes. The cells have small, inconspicuous nucleoli. One has villous cytoplasm and one is showing plasmacytoid differentiation. MGG × 960.

mantle-zone lymphoma is often difficult. The condition is characterized by very pleomorphic circulating lymphoma cells[13] (Fig. 4.10) of medium size but showing considerable variation. Some show inconspicuous nucleoli and some show nuclear indentations or clefts. Variable cytoplasmic basophilia occurs.

In the leukaemic phase of lymphoplasmacytoid lymphoma (Fig. 4.11), circulating cells resemble small lymphocytes but have some features of plasma cell differentiation such as cytoplasmic basophilia, a Golgi zone or an eccentric nucleus. Lymphoplasmacytoid lymphoma may manifest itself clinically as Waldenström's macroglobulinaemia or as cold haemagglutinin disease. SLVL can also be regarded as part of the spectrum of lymphoplasmacytoid lymphoma.

In the uncommon leukaemic phase of large cell lymphoma[14] (Fig. 4.12) cells are large and usually highly pleomorphic with prominent cytoplasmic basophilia. Nuclear chromatin may be diffuse or show some condensation. Nucleoli are common and may be conspicuous.

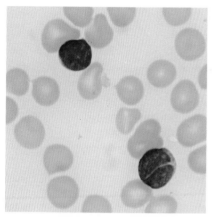

Fig. 4.9   PB film in leukaemic phase of follicular lymphoma. One cell is very small with scanty cytoplasm. The other is nucleolated and has a deep, narrow cleft. MGG × 960.

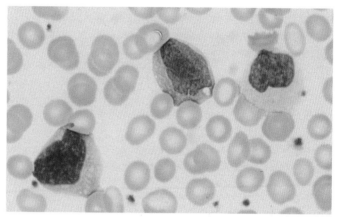

Fig. 4.10   PB film in intermediate (mantle-zone) lymphoma. The cells are markedly pleomorphic. MGG × 960.

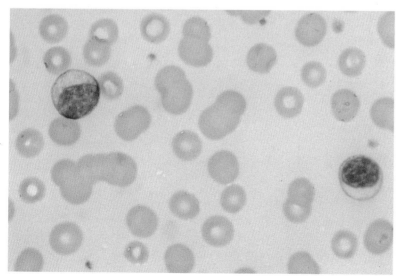

Fig. 4.11   PB film in Waldenström's macroglobulinaemia; this term describes a lymphoplasmacytoid lymphoma with production of large amount of monoclonal IgM. The blood film shows two plasmacytoid lymphocytes together with rouleaux and abnormal staining characteristics consequent on the high level of IgM. MGG × 960.

CELL MARKERS

The immunological phenotype of follicular lymphoma cells (Fig. 4.2) differs considerably from that of CLL cells. SmIg is strong, CD5 expression and MRFC are low and FMC7 expression is strong. CD10 may be expressed although expression is weaker than in cALL cells.

The immunological phenotype of the intermediate lymphoma cell is closer to that of the CLL cell in that CD5 is usually expressed and SmIg is usually of moderate intensity rather than strong, with μ and δ heavy chains predominating. MRFC are low, FMC7 and CD22 are usually expressed and CD10 is sometimes expressed.

The immunophenotype of lymphoplasmacytoid lymphoma cells is similar to that of plasma cells (see below) but FMC7 and CD22 may also be expressed.

Large cell lymphoma cells show a variable immunophenotype[15].

HISTOLOGY

When follicular lymphoma cells are present in the peripheral blood, the bone marrow is also infiltrated with characteristic cells. A bone marrow biopsy commonly shows broad-based paratrabecular infiltration although a diffuse pattern can also be seen. Although lymph nodes show a follicular pattern, follicles are often not apparent in the bone marrow biopsy.

In intermediate or mantle-zone lymphoma the bone marrow infiltration is diffuse. The lymph nodes show a diffuse infiltrate with sometimes a vague suggestion of nodularity. Lymphoma cells may infiltrate in the mantle zone around and within residual nonlymphomatous follicles.

CYTOGENETICS

A t(14;18)(q32;q21) translocation is very common in follicular lymphoma. Other lymphomas may show t(11;14), t(14;18), trisomy 12 or other anomalies.

Plasma cell leukaemia

The FAB group[1] have suggested that the term plasma cell leukaemia be confined to cases with *de novo* presentation in leukaemic phase, although similar circulating cells may be seen in the terminal phase of multiple myeloma. In *de novo* cases the patients have an acute illness, often with hepatosplenomegaly and sometimes also hypercalcaemia and renal failure.

MORPHOLOGY

Morphology varies considerably between cases. Some patients have mainly cells which resemble normal plasma cells with basophilic cytoplasm, a prominent Golgi zone and an eccentric nucleus (Fig. 4.13). Others have many lymphoplasmacytoid lymphocytes and only a minority of

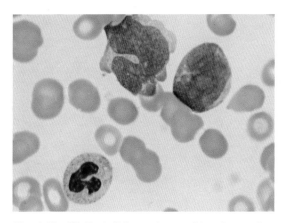

Fig. 4.12 PB film in B-lineage large cell lymphoma of centroblastic type. MGG × 960.

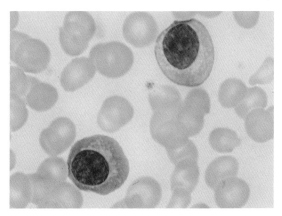

Fig. 4.13 PB film in plasma cell leukaemia. The malignant cells are identified as plasma cells by their eccentric nucleus and pale paranuclear area which is the Golgi zone. MGG × 960.

characteristic plasma cells. Yet others have more primitive cells with a higher nucleocytoplasmic ratio, a diffuse chromatin pattern, a prominent nucleolus and a less prominent Golgi zone; some such cases can be difficult to recognize as plasma cells by light microscopy alone.

MARKERS

In addition to the markers as shown in Fig. 4.2, positive reactions are found with McAb which are selective for plasma cells such as PCA-1 and BU11[1].

CYTOGENETICS

Plasma cell leukaemia shows cytogenetic abnormalities similar to those of multiple myeloma including t(11;14) (q13;q32) and other rearrangements with a 14q32 break-point and rearrangements of chromosomes 1 and 11.

CHRONIC LEUKAEMIAS OF T-LYMPHOCYTE LINEAGE

Chronic leukaemias of T-lymphocyte lineage are quite uncommon, constituting only a small proportion of chronic lymphoid leukaemias. Among them adult T-cell leukaemia/lymphoma is unique in being the only human leukaemia firmly linked to infection by a retrovirus. Chronic T-lineage leukaemias express one or more T-lymphocyte markers, commonly CD2, CD3, CD5 and either CD4 or CD8 (Figs. 4.14 and 4.15). The cells usually form rosettes with sheep red blood cells (ERFC). TdT, CD1 and CD38 are negative. In the T-lymphocyte lineage there is no readily available marker of mono-clonality equivalent to the SmIg of the B lymphocyte. Demonstration of clonality requires specialized techni-ques such as analysis of DNA to show rearrangement of one or more of the genes for the T-cell receptor β, γ or δ chains, or cytogenetic analysis. Clonality may, however, be inferred when a population of cells shows a uniform immunological phenotype. The FAB group have divided T-lineage lymphoproliferative disorders into four groups: T-CLL, T-PLL, adult T-cell leukaemia/lymphoma and the Sézary syndrome. They use the term T-CLL to indicate a proliferation of large granular lymphocytes and classify a leukaemia of cells morphologically resembling normal mature peripheral blood lymphocytes as small-cell variant of T-PLL rather than as T-CLL since they

have found that in such cases the ultrastructural and cytogenetic features resemble those of the typical case of T-PLL.

T chronic lymphocytic leukaemia

The FAB group use the term T chronic lymphocytic leukaemia (T-CLL)[1,16] to designate a condition which has previously been described under a variety of names including Tγ lymphoproliferative disorder and large granular lymphocyte (LGL) leukaemia[17,18]. The term chronic T-lymphocytosis has also been used to cover cases in whom clonality has not been demonstrated by genetic analysis or by the demonstration of a clonal cytogenetic abnormality and the neoplastic nature of the disorder is not certain; it is likely that many such cases are in fact leukaemic in nature. Some patients with T-CLL have little lymphadenopathy, splenomegaly or hepatomegaly and run a chronic course. Others have more prominent organomegaly and have a more acute course. A minority have skin infiltration or polyarthritis. Various cytopenias can occur, particularly neutropenia but also hypoplastic anaemia and thrombocytopenia. Some patients have hypogammaglobulinaemia.

MORPHOLOGY

The white cell count is usually only moderately increased. The abnormal lymphocytes are large with abundant, weakly basophilic cytoplasm containing small numbers of azurophilic granules ranging from fine to coarse (Fig. 4.16). Some cells are lacking in granules. The nucleus is round or oval and slightly eccentric with clumped chromatin and usually no visible nucleolus. Smear cells are not a feature.

CELL MARKERS

The most characteristic phenotype is CD2, CD3, CD8 and CD57 (Leu 7) positive and CD4, CD11b and CD16 negative (Fig. 4.15). CD7 is sometimes positive. Recep-tors for Fcγ are also commonly present. CD57 positivity, which is useful in distinguishing T-CLL from other disorders of T lymphocytes, is characteristic of natural killer cells which may also have LGL morphology. A minority of cases of T-CLL have markers rarely seen in normal peripheral blood large granular lymphocytes with

Cluster designation	Representative McAb	Specificity within haemopoietic lineage
SOME MONOCLONAL ANTIBODIES USED IN THE CHARACTERIZATION OF CHRONIC LYMPHOID LEUKAEMIAS OF T LINEAGE		
CD2, CD3, CD5, CD7	see Fig. 3.2	E-receptor and other T-cell associated antigens (see Fig. 3.2)
CD4	OKT4, T4, Leu3	common and late thymocytes, subset of mature T cells (among which are many cells which are functionally helper/inducer) which recognize antigens in a Class II context, monocytes
CD8	OKT8, T8, Leu2	common and late thymocytes, subset of mature T cells (among which are many cells which are functionally cytotoxic/suppressor) which recognize antigens in a Class I context
CD11b	Mo1, OKM1, Leu 15	C3bi receptor: monocytes, granulocytes, natural killer (NK) cells
CD16	Leu 11b	FcRIII: NK cells, granulocytes, macrophages
CD56	Leu 19, NKH1	natural killer cells, activated lymphocytes
CD57	Leu 7	HNK1: natural killer cells, T cells, B-cell subset
CD25, CD38, anti-Ia		see Fig. 4.1

Fig. 4.14 Some monoclonal antibodies used in the characterization of chronic leukaemias of T-lineage.

Marker	T-CLL	T-PLL	ATLL	Sézary syndrome
IMMUNOPHENOTYPE OF CHRONIC T-CELL LEUKAEMIAS				
ERFC/CD2	++	++	++	++
CD3	++	+	++	++
CD5	−	++	++	++
CD7	−	++	−	−
CD4	−	+	++	++
CD8	++	−/+	−	−
CD25	−	−	++	−

The incidence with which a marker is positive in $>$ 30 percent of cells in a particular leukaemia is indicated as follows: ++ 80–100 percent; + 40–80 percent; −/+ 10–40 percent; − 0–9 percent.

T-CLL, T-cell chronic lymphocytic leukaemia (large granular lymphocyte leukaemia); T-PLL, T-cell prolymphocytic leukaemia; ATLL, adult T-cell leukaemia/lymphoma; ERFC, E rosette forming cells.

Fig. 4.15 Characteristic immunological phenotype in chronic leukaemias of T-lineage. Modified from Bennett et al[1].

coexpression of CD4 and natural killer (NK) markers or a pure NK phenotype. They include: (i) CD3+, CD8+, CD11b+; (ii) CD3+, CD4+, CD16+; (iii) CD3+, CD4+, CD11b+ and (iv) CD3−, CD4−, CD8− but CD11b+, CD16+, CD56+ or CD57+. The less usual phenotypes tend to be associated with more rapidly progressive disease.

HISTOLOGY

Bone marrow infiltration is minor in the early stages. It may be focal or interstitial.

CYTOGENETICS

A number of clonal cytogenetic abnormalities have been described in T-CLL but no consistent association has been recognized.

T-prolymphocytic leukaemia

Cases of T-prolymphocytic leukaemia (T-PLL)[1,19] resemble B-PLL in presenting most commonly with marked

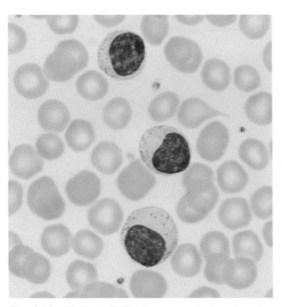

Fig. 4.16 PB film in T-CLL (large granular lymphocyte leukaemia). The cells have abundant weakly basophilic cytoplasm containing prominent azurophilic granules. MGG × 960.

splenomegaly and a high white cell count. They differ in that lymphadenopathy, skin lesions and serous effusions may also be present. The clinical course is aggressive.

MORPHOLOGY

In about half of the cases of T-PLL the morphology is similar to that of B-PLL although the nuclear outline may be more irregular. In other patients cells are smaller with a higher nucleocytoplasmic ratio (Fig. 4.17). Cytoplasm is usually deeply basophilic. In about one-quarter of patients the cells are small and the nucleolus is not easily detectable on light microscopy. It is likely that this latter small-cell variant of T-PLL has in the past often been designated T-CLL rather than T-PLL. The FAB group justify their classification by the observations that patients with the small-cell variant have a prominent nucleolus on ultrastructural examination, have the same clinical course as other patients and show the same cytogenetic abnormality (see below).

CELL MARKERS

Most cases of T-PLL are CD2, CD3, CD5, CD7 and CD4 positive and CD8 negative[1] (Fig. 4.15). The remainder are negative for CD4 and positive for CD8 or coexpress these two markers. A minority of cases are CD25 positive. CD7 positivity helps to distinguish T-PLL from other disorders of mature T cells.

HISTOLOGY

The bone marrow infiltration is usually interstitial or diffuse although an interstitial/nodular pattern has also been reported. Lymph node infiltration is diffuse and mainly paracortical. The splenic red pulp is diffusely infiltrated with the white pulp being obliterated.

CYTOGENETICS

About two-thirds of cases of T-PLL show inv(14)(q11; q32)[20]. Some patients with and others without inv(14) show translocations involving 14q11, the site of the TCR α gene. Other defects seen include trisomy 8q consequent on t(8:8) or i(8q) and translocations with a breakpoint at 7q35, the site of the TCR β gene.

Adult T cell leukaemia/lymphoma

Adult T cell leukaemia/lymphoma (ATLL)[1,21,22] occurs in adults who are carriers of the type-C retrovirus, HTLV-1; the provirus DNA is clonally integrated into the DNA of the neoplastic cells. Presentation is with lymphadenopathy, bone and skin lesions, hypercalcaemia and usually circulating lymphoma cells. Some patients have hepatomegaly or splenomegaly or infiltration of other organs. Prognosis is generally poor but some patients have a subacute or smouldering disease. Distribution of the disease relates to areas where the virus is endemic. Cases were first recognized in Japan, and subsequently in the Caribbean, in the southern United States and in West Indian immigrants to the UK and other countries. Smaller numbers of cases have been reported from Central and West Africa, South America and Taiwan.

MORPHOLOGY

The number of circulating lymphoma cells is very variable. The morphology is distinctive (Fig. 4.18). Cells vary greatly in size and form. Most cells have condensed and relatively homogeneous nuclear chromatin with nucleoli being infrequent and small. A minority of cells are blastic with basophilic cytoplasm. Some cells have convoluted nuclei which may resemble Sézary cells, while many are polylobated with some nuclei resembling clover leaves.

CELL MARKERS

ATLL cells form E-rosettes and are usually positive for CD2, CD3, CD5, CD4, and CD25[1] (Fig. 4.15). Positivity for CD25 helps to distinguish ATLL from other T-cell disorders which are usually CD25 negative. A minority of cases have been reported to be positive for Ia, CD7 or CD38.

HISTOLOGY

The bone marrow may initially be normal or may show diffuse infiltration which becomes heavier as the white cell count rises. Lymph nodes show diffuse infiltration, either paracortical or effacing nodal architecture. Infiltration in the skin is perivascular or diffuse in the middle and upper dermis; some cases show epidermotropism with formation of intraepidermal lymphoid infiltrates known as Pautrier's microabscesses, formerly thought to be confined to the Sézary syndrome.

CYTOGENETICS

A variety of chromosomal abnormalities have been described in ATLL, most commonly trisomy 12, 6q− and rearrangements with breakpoints at 7p14 or 15, 14q11−13 or 14q32[23]. Rearrangements of 1p32−36 and 5q11−13 may be preferentially associated with ATLL.

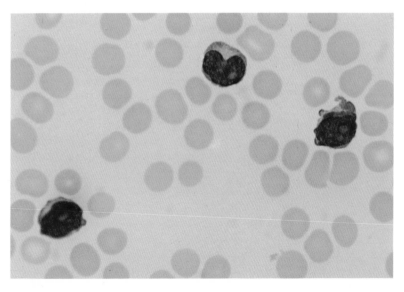

Fig. 4.17 PB film in T-PLL. In this case the nuclei are more irregular and the nucleoli are less conspicuous than in B-PLL. MGG × 960.

Sézary syndrome

The Sézary syndrome is characterized by circulating lymphoma cells and a skin infiltration which manifests itself clinically as generalized exfoliative erythroderma. The Sézary syndrome is closely related to mycosis fungoides in which circulating lymphoma cells are not necessarily seen; in some cases of mycosis fungoides the skin manifestations are similar to those of the Sézary syndrome but in other cases the skin shows plaques, nodules or fungating tumours. The term cutaneous T-cell lymphoma has been used to embrace both the Sézary syndrome and mycosis fungoides, together with a number of other T-cell lymphomas in which the skin is the primary organ involved.

MORPHOLOGY

Sézary cells[1] (Fig. 4.19) may be either large or small, and one or other form usually predominates in an individual patient. Large Sézary cells are similar in size to a neutrophil or a monocyte, with a high nucleocytoplasmic ratio and a round or oval nucleus with densely condensed chromatin, a grooved surface and usually no detectable nucleolus. Small Sézary cells are similar in size to a normal small lymphocyte, with a high nucleocytoplasmic ratio and a dense nucleus with a grooved surface and no visible nucleolus. Some cells show a ring of cytoplasmic vacuoles which PAS-staining shows to be due to the presence of glycogen. Small Sézary cells in particular may be difficult to identify on light microscopy. Electron

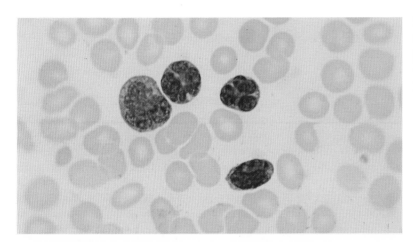

Fig. 4.18   PB film in ATLL. Cells are pleomorphic with polylobulated nuclei, one of which resembles a clover leaf. MGG × 960.

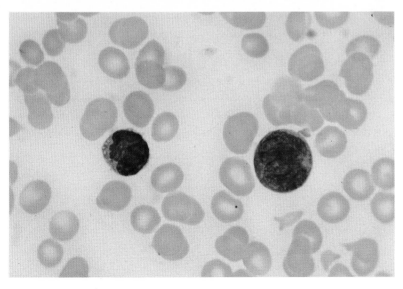

Fig. 4.19   PB film in Sézary syndrome. Both cells have convoluted nuclei. The smaller one has inconspicuous cytoplasmic vacuoles. MGG × 960.

microscopy can be very useful since it reveals the highly complex, convoluted nucleus which is not so readily detectable by light microscopy.

CELL MARKERS

Sézary cells are characteristically positive for CD2, CD3, CD5 and CD4, and negative for CD8[1] (Fig. 4.15).

HISTOLOGY

The bone marrow is usually either normal or minimally infiltrated with a diffuse pattern of infiltration. Skin infiltration is in the upper dermis, particularly around the skin appendages, and within the epidermis forming Pautrier's microabscesses. Epidermotropism and Pautrier's microabscesses are characteristic of Sézary syndrome and mycosis fungoides but are not pathognomic of these conditions since they have now been observed also in a number of cases of ATLL.

CYTOGENETICS

A great variety of cytogenetic abnormalities have been reported in Sézary syndrome without any consistent association being apparent. Karyotypes are often highly complex and polyploid cells are not uncommon.

T-cell non-Hodgkin's lymphoma

Rarely leukaemia occurs as a manifestation of T-lineage large cell lymphoma, either at presentation or during the course of the illness. Morphologically the cells cannot be distinguished from those of B-lineage large cell lymphoma[14] so study of immunological markers is essential for diagnosis. Although the phenotype is that of a mature T cell, there is no consistent pattern and immunophenotypes rarely seen in normal peripheral blood T-cells are common[15].

DISCUSSION OF THE FAB PROPOSALS FOR A CLASSIFICATION OF THE CHRONIC LYMPHOID LEUKAEMIAS

There is clearly a need for more precise diagnosis and an improved classification of the chronic lymphoid leukaemias, since conditions which differ in their prognosis and their response to therapy have in the past not been differentiated from one another. This is particularly true of the chronic leukaemias of T lineage since 'T chronic lymphocytic leukaemia' has been used as a general term to cover proliferations of large granular lymphocytes, small-cell variant of T-PLL and other ill-defined conditions[24]. Interpretation of reports of cytogenetic abnormalities in T-lineage leukaemias is made difficult by the frequency of inadequate descriptions of the characteristics of cases and by the lack of any agreed terminology. The proposals of the FAB group[1] are an attempt to provide such an agreed terminology. Since they have been only recently promulgated there has not as yet been time for other groups to assess or apply this classification. This chapter is therefore predominantly an explanation of the classification, based to a large extent on the publications of the FAB group and their co-workers rather than a critical analysis of its application. More time is needed to see if the classification wins general acceptance. One point which is likely to give rise to discussion is whether T-CLL is the best term to adopt to describe a proliferation of large granular lymphocytes since it is likely that the term will continue to be used with other meanings, and without the sense in which it is used always being clear. For this reason 'large granular lymphocyte leukaemia' although more cumbersome might be preferable. The latter term has now been recommended by the MIC group[25]

REFERENCES

1. Bennett JM, Catovsky D, Daniel M-T, Flandrin G, Galton DAG, Gralnick HR & Sultan C (1989) Proposals for the classification of chronic (mature) B and T lymphoid leukaemias. *Journal of Clinical Pathology*, **42**, 567–584.

2. Lampert I & Thompson I (1988). In *Chronic lymphocytic leukemia*. Edited by A Polliack & D Catovsky. Harwood Academic Publishers, London.

3. Lampert I, Catovsky D, Marsh GW, Child JA & Galton DAG (1980) The histopathology of prolymphocytic leukaemia with particular reference to the spleen: a comparison with chronic lymphocytic leukaemia. *Histopathology*, **4**, 3–19.

4. Enno A, Catovsky D, O'Brien M, Cherchi M, Kumaran TO & Galton DAG (1979) "Prolymphocytoid" transformation of chronic lymphocytic leukaemia. *British Journal of Haematology*, **41**, 9–18.

5. Melo JV, Catovsky D & Galton DAG (1986) The relationship between chronic lymphocytic leukaemia and prolymphocytic leukaemia. I. Clinical and laboratory features of 300 patients and characterisation of an intermediate group. *British Journal of Haematology*, **63**, 377–387.

6. Galton DAG, Goldman JM, Wiltshaw E, Catovsky D, Henry K & Goldenberg GJ (1974) Prolymphocytic leukaemia. *British Journal of Haematology*, **27**, 7–23.

7. Brito-Babapulle V, Pittman S, Melo JV, Pomfret M & Catovsky D (1987) Cytogenetic studies on prolymphocytic leukemia I. B-cell prolymphocytic leukemia. *Hematologic Pathology*, **1**, 27–33.

8. Cawley JC, Burns GF & Hayhoe FGH (1980) A chronic lymphoproliferative disorder with distinctive features: a distinct variant of hairy cell leukemia. *Leukemia Research*, **4**, 547–559.

9. Matutes E, Mulligan S, Sainati L, Dearden C & Catovsky D (1989) A variant form of hairy cell leukemia resistant to alpha-interferon. *Blood*, **74**, Supplement 237a.

10. Bain BJ, Morilla R, Monard S, Kokai Y & Catovsky D (1990) Spectrum of reactivity with three monoclonal antibodies – MHM6 (CD23), L30 (CD24) and UCHB1 – in B cell leukaemias. Submitted for publication.

11. Melo JV, Hegde U, Parreira A, Thompson I, Lampert IA & Catovsky D (1987) Splenic B lymphoma with circulating villous lymphocytes: differential diagnosis of B cell leukaemias with large spleens. *Journal of Clinical Pathology*, **40**, 329–342.

12. Melo JV, Robinson DSF, de Oliviera MP, Thompson IW, Lampert IA, Ng JP, Galton DAG & Catovsky D (1988) Morphology and immunology of circulating cells in leukaemic phase of follicular lymphoma. *Journal of Clinical Pathology*, **41**, 951–959.

13. de Oliveira M, Jaffe E & Catovsky D (1989) Leukaemic phase of mantle zone (intermediate) lymphoma: its characterisation in 11 cases. *Journal of Clinical Pathology*, **42**, 962–972.

14. Bain BJ, Matutes E, Robinson D, Lampert AI, Brito-Babapulle V & Catovsky D (1990) Leukaemia as a manifestation of large cell lymphoma. I Clinical, cytological and ultrastructural features. In preparation.

15. Matutes E, Bain BJ & Catovsky D (1990) Leukaemia as a manifestation of large cell lymphoma. II Immunological and molecular biological features. In preparation.

16. Matutes E, Brito-Babapulle V, Worner I, Sainati L, Foroni L & Catovsky D (1988) T-cell chronic lymphocytic leukaemia: the spectrum of mature T-cell disorders. *Nouvelle Revue Française d'Hématologie*, **30**, 347–351.

17. Reynolds CW & Foon KA (1984) Tγ-lymphoproliferative disease and related disorders in humans and experimental animals: a review of the clinical, cellular and functional characteristics. *Blood*, **64**, 1146.

18. Oshimi K (1988) Granular lymphocyte proliferative disorders: report of 12 cases and review of the literature. *Leukemia*, **2**, 617–627.

19. Matutes E, Garcia Talavera J, O'Brien M & Catovsky D (1986) The morphological spectrum of T-prolymphocytic leukaemia. *British Journal of Haematology*, **41**, 111–124.

20. Brito-Babapulle V, Pomfret M, Matutes E & Catovsky D (1987) Cytogenetic studies on prolymphocytic leukemia. II. T cell prolymphocytic leukemia. *Blood*, **70**, 926–931.

21. Uchiyama T, Yodoi J, Sagawa K, Takatsuki K & Uchino H (1977) Adult T-cell leukemia: clinical and hematological features of 16 cases. *Blood*, **50**, 481–492.

22. Catovsky D, Greaves MF, Rose M, Galton DAG, Goolden AWG, McCluskey DR, White JM, Lampert I, Bourikas G, Ireland R, Bridges JM, Blattner WA & Gallo RC (1982) Adult T-cell lymphoma – leukaemia in Blacks from the West Indies. *Lancet*, **i**, 639–643.

23. Fifth international workshop on chromosomes in leukemia-lymphoma (1988) Correlation of chromosome abnormalities with histologic and immunologic characteristics in non-Hodgkin's lymphoma and adult T-cell leukemia lymphoma. *Blood*, **70**, 1554–1564.

24. Knowles DM (1986) The human T-cell leukemias: clinical, cytomorphologic, immunophenotypic, and genotypic characteristics. *Human Pathology*, **17**, 14–33.

25. Bennett J, Juliusson G & Mecucci C (1990) A conference on the Morphologic, Immunologic, and Cytogenetic classification of the chronic (mature) B and T lymphoid leukaemias (MIC IV). *British Journal of Haematology*, **74**, 240.

chapter five

OTHER LEUKAEMIAS

The FAB group have not yet proposed a classification for the chronic myeloid leukaemias. For completeness, these and several other rare forms of leukaemia which are not included in the FAB classification will be briefly described here.

CHRONIC GRANULOCYTIC LEUKAEMIA

Chronic granulocytic leukaemia (CGL) is predominantly a disease of adults. The usual clinical presentation is with splenomegaly, hepatomegaly, symptoms of anaemia, and systemic symptoms such as sweating and weight loss.

The usual haematological features are anaemia and leucocytosis with a very characteristic differential count. The two predominant cell types in the peripheral blood are the myelocyte and the mature neutrophil[1] (Fig. 5.1). More immature granulocyte precursors are present but promyelocytes are fewer than myelocytes and blasts are fewer than promyelocytes. Almost all patients have an absolute basophilia, and about 80 percent have eosinophilia. The absolute monocyte count is increased, but not in proportion to mature neutrophils, and the percentage of monocytes is almost always less than 3 percent. Occasional nucleated red blood cells and occasional megakaryocyte nuclei may be present. The platelet count is most often normal or somewhat elevated but is low in about 5 percent of cases. Rarely the haemoglobin concentration is elevated. The NAP score is low in about 95 percent of patients. Bone marrow findings are of much less importance than the peripheral blood features in the differential diagnosis of the chronic myeloid leukaemias. The bone marrow in CGL is intensely hyper-cellular with marked granulocytic hyperplasia (Fig. 5.2) and with the myeloid:erythroid (M:E) ratio being greater than 10:1. Megakaryocytes are increased in number and, on average, they are smaller and their lobe count is lower than those of normal megakaryocytes. Rarely the bone marrow is fibrotic at presentation.

CGL is associated with a characteristic chromosome abnormality, t(9;22)(q34;q11) with derivative chromosomes 9q+ and 22q−, the latter being known as the Philadelphia (Ph) chromosome. The translocation results in the juxtaposition of the sequences in the breakpoint cluster region of chromosome 22 with the cellular onco-gene, c-*abl*, from chromosome 9 to form a hybrid gene (bcr-*abl*) thought to be important in the causation of CGL. The 9;22 translocation occurs in a multipotent stem cell so that the clone of cells with this abnormality includes the granulocyte, monocyte, erythroid and megakaryocyte lineages, and also some precursors of at least B lymphocytes and possibly T lymphocytes. The Ph chromosome is found in about 95 percent of typical cases of CGL. In other cases a Ph chromosome is formed but is masked, for example by translocation to a third chromosome. Some further cases do not have a detect-able Ph chromosome, but nevertheless are clinically and morphologically indistinguishable from CGL. They should be classified as Ph-negative CGL. In the great majority of such cases a fusion gene with sequences from chromosomes 9 and 22 has been formed even though no translocation is detectable by microscopical examination of the chromosomes. Other cases of chronic myeloid leukaemia not only are Ph-negative but differ morphologically from Ph-positive CGL; they are better classified as atypical Ph-negative chronic myeloid leukaemia (see below). CGL has also been designated chronic myeloid

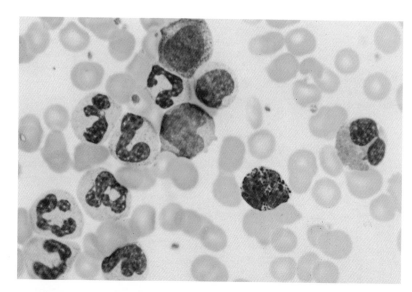

Fig. 5.1 PB film of a patient with chronic granulocytic leukaemia showing two promyelocytes, a myelocyte, an eosinophil, a basophil and numerous neutrophils and band forms. MGG × 960.

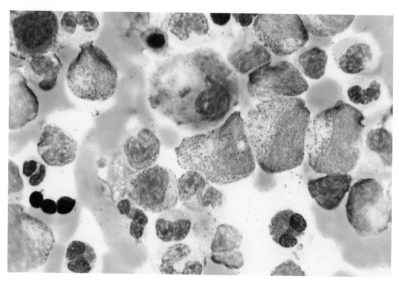

Fig. 5.2 BM film of a patient with chronic granulocytic leukaemia showing granulocytic hyperplasia and a phagocyte containing cellular debris. MGG × 384.

leukaemia, but it seems preferable to use the former term for the Ph-positive disease, and conditions morphologically indistinguishable from it, so that the term chronic myeloid leukaemia can be used in a more general sense, in a manner analogous to the use of the term acute myeloid leukaemia.

CGL terminates in blast crisis, that is by transformation into a more acute leukaemia. This may be myeloid, lymphoid or biphenotypic/bilineage. Myeloid transformation may be mixed or may be predominantly myeloblastic, monoblastic, myelomonocytic, eosinophilic, basophilic and/or mast cell, hypergranular promyelocytic,

megakaryoblastic or erythroid. Acute myelofibrosis occasionally develops, sometimes with associated osteosclerosis; this is most commonly associated with megakaryocytic/megakaryoblastic transformations. In contrast to *de novo* acute myeloid leukaemia, Auer rods are rarely seen in myeloid blast crisis. Lymphoid blast crisis is usually B lineage but occasionally T lineage. B-lineage lymphoid blast crisis may be early precursor B cell or have a common ALL or a pre-B phenotype. Biphenotypic/bilineage leukaemias are relatively much more common in CGL in transformation than in *de novo* acute leukaemias.

Prior to blast transformation, CGL may enter an accelerated phase with a decreasing clinical response to therapy and with refractory leucocytosis, basophilia and anaemia. Myelodysplastic features may be seen including ring sideroblasts, the acquired Pelger–Huët anomaly of neutrophils or eosinophils, and small round nucleus (SRN) megakaryocytes.

ATYPICAL (PH-NEGATIVE) CHRONIC MYELOID LEUKAEMIA

Cases of atypical chronic myeloid leukaemia (CML) usually present with splenomegaly and symptoms of anaemia. Patients are on average 15 to 20 years older than those with CGL.

There is a leucocytosis with an increase of both neutrophils and their precursors, but monocytes are also prominent while eosinophilia and basophilia are less common than in CGL[2] (Fig. 5.3). On average the white cell count is lower and anaemia and thrombocytopenia are more common. Morphological abnormalities, which are not a feature of CGL, are common in atypical CML. Neutrophils may be hypogranular or have nuclei of abnormal shape. Some neutrophils showing the acquired Pelger–Huët anomaly may be present. Promyelocytes, myelocytes and metamyelocytes are sometimes hypogranular. Monocytes may be immature. The NAP score is commonly decreased and in a minority of patients is increased. The bone marrow findings reflect those in the peripheral blood. There is granulocytic hyperplasia but, in contrast to CGL, the M:E ratio is usually less than 10:1. In comparison with CGL, basophil and eosinophil precursors are less often increased whereas monocyte precursors are sometimes more prominent (Fig. 5.4). Megakaryocytes are reduced in about one-third of patients. Blasts may be somewhat increased but are less than 30 percent.

Atypical CML needs to be distinguished from chronic myelomonocytic leukaemia. This is most readily done on the basis of the much higher percentage of circulating granulocyte precursors in atypical CML (see page 53). The total white cell count is also higher than in the majority of patients with CMML. It can also sometimes be difficult to distinguish atypical CML from CGL presenting with dysplastic features and already in early transformation. Cytogenetic and molecular analysis are necessary to make the distinction reliably.

Atypical CML, like CGL, terminates in blast crisis. This is usually a myeloid crisis but occasional lymphoid blast crises have been observed[3] suggesting that this condition, like CGL, may arise in a pluripotent stem cell.

A number of clonal chromosomal abnormalities have been reported. No consistent association has been recognized although trisomy 8 may be most common. Genetic rearrangement with production of a bcr-*abl* fusion gene has been reported in rare cases of atypical CML as well as in Ph-negative CGL[4].

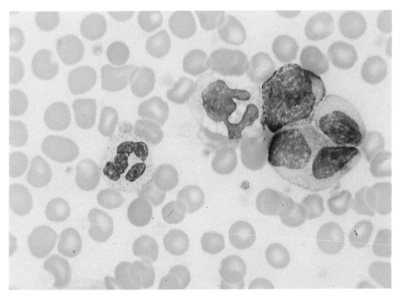

Fig. 5.3 PB film of a patient with atypical (Philadelphia-negative) chronic myeloid leukaemia showing a neutrophil, a monocyte, a promyelocyte and two myelocytes, one of which is binucleate. MGG × 960.

CHRONIC NEUTROPHILIC LEUKAEMIA

Chronic neutrophilic leukaemia is a rare condition, largely confined to the elderly, characterized by anaemia, spleno-megaly and sometimes hepatomegaly. The neutrophil count is markedly increased but the peripheral blood shows few granulocyte precursors (Fig. 5.5). Toxic granulation, Döhle bodies and ring-shaped neutrophil nuclei may be present. Typical myelodysplastic features are not usually seen but a variant has been described in

which they are prominent[5]. The NAP score is usually high. A variety of clonal cytogenetic abnormalities have been reported. The Ph chromosome is not present and in the few cases reported the fusion bcr-*abl* gene was not present. Blastic transformation of chronic neutrophilic leukaemia is uncommon, although it appears to be much more common in patients with prominent myelodys-plastic features whose disease may in fact be closer to the myelodysplastic syndromes than to chronic neutrophilic leukaemia as usually recognized.

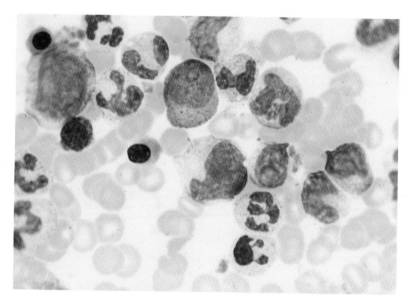

Fig. 5.4 BM film of the same patient as shown in Fig. 5.3 showing granulocytic hyperplasia with dysplastic features and several cells of monocyte lineage. MGG × 960.

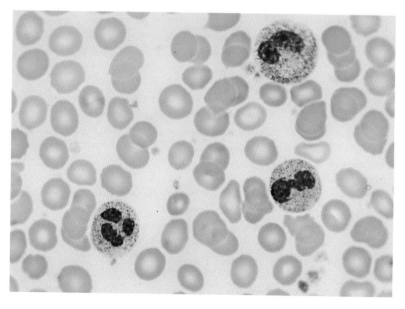

Fig. 5.5 PB film of a patient with neutrophilic leukaemia showing an increase of mature neutrophils which show toxic granulation. MGG × 960.

JUVENILE CHRONIC MYELOID LEUKAEMIA

Juvenile chronic myeloid leukaemia[6] is mainly a disease of children of less than five years of age. The usual clinical features are anaemia with splenomegaly and sometimes hepatomegaly, lymphadenopathy or a rash. The peripheral blood shows neutrophilia and prominent monocytosis. Granulocyte precursors are sometimes present. Anaemia, thrombocytopenia and circulating nucleated red blood cells are common. The bone marrow is hypercellular with granulocytic hyperplasia and sometimes an increase also in monocyte numbers. Blasts are often somewhat elevated.

Juvenile chronic myeloid leukaemia is associated with reversion to some characteristics of fetal erythropoiesis. The haemoglobin F level and the expression of i antigen are increased while the percentage of haemoglobin A_2, the carbonic anhydrase activity and the expression of I antigen are reduced.

The NAP score is variable. The concentration of Ig is increased in about 50 percent of cases. A variety of clonal chromosomal abnormalities have been described. Some patients undergo blastic transformation but even those who do not, show a poor prognosis.

Juvenile chronic myeloid leukaemia is readily distinguished on haematological grounds from CGL, which in any event is very rare in young children. It can also be distinguished from the myelodysplastic/myeloproliferative disorder of children associated with monosomy 7 (see page 47). If cytogenetic studies are not readily available the concentration of haemoglobin F has been proposed as a useful way of making the distinction, with a level of 15 percent or more suggesting that the diagnosis is juvenile chronic myeloid leukaemia.

BASOPHILIC LEUKAEMIA

Cases of leukaemia showing basophilic differentiation with 30 percent or more of blast cells in the bone marrow are included in the FAB classification of acute leukaemia; they generally fall into the M2Baso or M4Baso categories but some are best categorized as M0Baso (see page 29). Cases of basophilic leukaemia with fewer blast cells generally have a chronic course. The majority have been demonstrated to have the Ph chromosome[7] and are best regarded as a variant of CGL. Patients with basophilic leukaemia may have signs and symptoms consequent on histamine excess[8].

MAST CELL LEUKAEMIA

Mast cell leukaemia occurs either as a *de novo* leukaemia or as the terminal phase of systemic mastocytosis. Since the mast cell is derived from a myeloid stem cell, systemic mastocytosis can be regarded as a myeloproliferative disorder; it terminates in acute myeloid leukaemia (of various FAB subtypes) more commonly than it terminates in mast cell leukaemia.

The usual clinical features of mast cell leukaemia are anaemia, hepatomegaly, splenomegaly, lymphadenopathy and symptoms of histamine excess including peptic ulceration[8]. The clinical course is that of an acute leukaemia. The peripheral blood shows mast cells (Fig. 5.6) which are often immature or morphologically abnormal with hypogranularity of lobulated nuclei. The bone marrow is hypercellular and infiltrated by mast cells. In systemic mastocytosis there is often peripheral blood and bone marrow eosinophilia and the bone marrow biopsy may show myelofibrosis and osteosclerosis; these features are not at all common in *de novo* mast cell leukaemia. Mast cells stain metachromatically with a Giemsa stain and they are therefore much more readily detected with this stain than with an H&E stain. Their presence can be confirmed by a positive CAE reaction and metachromatic staining with toluidine blue or Alcian blue.

EOSINOPHILIC LEUKAEMIA

Cases of leukaemia with eosinophilic differentiation and with 30 percent or more blasts in the bone marrow are included in the FAB classification of acute leukaemia; they are usually M2Eo or M4Eo, sometimes associated with t(8;21) and inv(16) respectively. Eosinophil proliferation is also sometimes associated with ALL. In many such cases it is likely that the eosinophilia is reactive and in some cases it has been demonstrated that the eosinophils lack a cytogenetic abnormality which is present in the leukaemic clone. In a few cases, however, a cytogenetic abnormality has been demonstrated in eosinophils suggesting that they are leukaemic and that the leukaemia is in fact bilineage rather than ALL.

Patients with eosinophilic leukaemia usually present with anaemia, thrombocytopenia, hepatomegaly, splenomegaly, lymphadenopathy and signs and symptoms of damage to the heart and other tissues by the contents of eosinophil granules. Blasts may be increased in the blood or bone marrow and eosinophils commonly show morphological abnormalities such as vacuolation and degranulation. Survival in those with fewer than 30 percent bone marrow blasts is variable, but often quite short.

A particular problem occurs in establishing the diagnosis of eosinophilic leukaemia in patients with a marked proliferation of mature eosinophils but with no increase of blast cells. The differential diagnosis is between reactive eosinophilia, leukaemia, and the idiopathic hypereosinophilic syndrome. The nature of the latter condition is not certain. Although it may well be a chronic myeloproliferative disorder, it has rarely been demonstrated that the eosinophils are clonal or neoplastic. Marked eosinophilia and the presence of morphological abnormalities in eosinophils are of little use in confirming the diagnosis of leukaemia since they may occur also in reactive eosinophilia and in the idiopathic hypereosinophilic syndrome. The demonstration of a clonal cytogenetic abnormality can be regarded as confirmatory. If there is neither an increase in blast cells nor a cytogenetic abnormality, the noncommital diagnosis of idiopathic hypereosinophilic syndrome is preferable, although some cases which are so classified may subsequently transform into acute myeloid leukaemia, providing evidence that the disorder was leukaemic, or at least, preleukaemic from the outset. A number of chromosomal abnormalities have been observed in eosinophilic leukaemia, including trisomy 8, i(17q), t(10;11) and abnormalities of 12p.

TRANSIENT ABNORMAL MYELOPOIESIS OF DOWN'S SYNDROME

Neonates with Down's syndrome have been observed to have a condition which closely resembles acute leukaemia but which resolves spontaneously, to be later followed, in some but not all cases, by acute leukaemia which does not resolve. This phenomenon has been regarded as a leukaemoid reaction but since a number of children have been observed to have a proliferating cytogenetically abnormal clone it seems likely that it is really a transient leukaemia. These cases have hepatosplenomegaly, anaemia and sometimes thrombocytopenia with large numbers of blasts in the blood and marrow (Figs. 5.7 and 5.8). Some babies die as a result of the bone marrow dysfunction. The abnormal cells are often megakaryoblasts but sometimes have features of primitive erythroid cells or of basophiloblasts[9]. The acute leukaemia which follows in some cases after an interval of months or even years is not necessarily of the same morphological type and may show a different cytogenetic abnormality. These apparent leukaemias may be described morphologically according to the FAB classification but they should not be grouped with other cases of acute leukaemia in neonates since the prognosis differs and, in view of the high probability of spontaneous remission, it is generally considered that only supportive treatment is indicated.

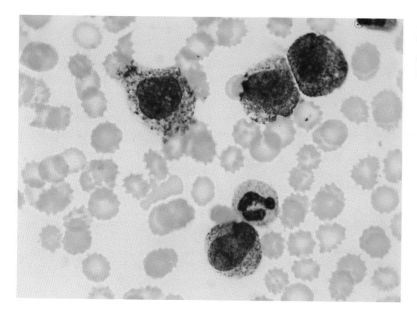

Fig. 5.6 PB film of a patient with mast cell leukaemia showing a neutrophil and four mastocytes. MGG × 960.

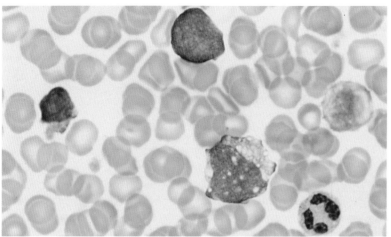

Fig. 5.7 PB film of a neonate with transient abnormal myelopoiesis of Down's syndrome showing a neutrophil, a giant platelet, an unidentifiable abnormal cell, a blast cell and a micromegakaryocyte which is similar in size to a lymphocyte. The blast cells were demonstrated to be megakaryoblasts by immunological markers. MGG × 960.

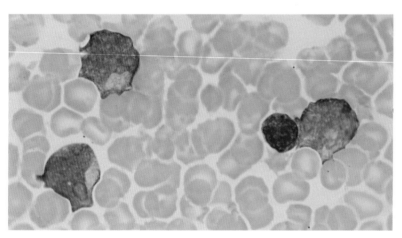

Fig. 5.8 BM film of the same patient as shown in Fig. 5.7 showing a lymphocyte and three pleomorphic blasts. × 960.

REFERENCES

1. Spiers ASD, Bain BJ & Turner JE (1977) The peripheral blood in chronic granulocytic leukaemia. *Scandinavian Journal of Haematology*, **18**, 25–38.

2. Kantarjian HM, Keating MJ, Walters RS, McCredie KB, Smith TL, Talpaz M, Beran M, Cork A, Trujillo JM & Freireich EJ (1986) Clinical and prognostic features of philadelphia chromosome-negative chronic myelogenous leukemia. *Cancer*, **58**, 2023–2030.

3. Hughes A, McVerry BA, Walter H, Bradstock KF, Hoffbrand AV & Janossy G (1981) Heterogeneous blast crises in Philadelphia negative chronic granulocytic leukaemia. *British Journal of Haematology*, **46**, 563–569.

4. Dreazen O, Klisak I, Rassool F, Goldman JM, Sparkes RS & Gale RP (1987) Do oncogenes determine clinical features in chronic myeloid leukaemia? *Lancet*, **i**, 1402–1405.

5. Zoumbos NC, Symeonidis A & Kourakli-Symeonidis A (1989) Chronic neutrophilic leukemia with dysplastic features: a new variant of myelodysplastic syndromes? *Acta Haematologica*, **82**, 156–160.

6. Castro-Malapina H, Schaison G, Passe S, Pasquier A, Berger R, Bayle-Weisgerber C, Miller D, Seligman M & Bernard J (1984) Subacute and chronic myelomonocytic leukaemia in children (Juvenile chronic myeloid leukaemia). *Cancer*, **54**, 675–686.

7. Goh K-o & Anderson FW (1979) Cytogenetic studies in basophilic chronic myelocytic leukemia. *Archives of Pathology and Laboratory Medicine*, **103**, 288–290.

8. Travis WD, Li C-Y, Hoagland HC, Travis LB & Banks PM (1986) Mast cell leukemia: report of a case and review of the literature. *Mayo Clinic Proceedings*, **61**, 957–966.

9. Bessho F, Hayashi Y, Hayashi Y & Ohga K (1986) Ultrastructural studies of peripheral blood of neonates with Down's syndrome and transient abnormal myelopoiesis. *American Journal of Pathology*, **88**, 627–633.

APPENDIX

The members of the French–American–British (FAB) cooperative group

J.M. Bennett
University of Rochester Cancer Centre
University of Rochester School of
Medicine and Dentistry, Rochester,
New York, USA.

D. Catovsky
Department of Academic Haematology
and Cytogenetics, Royal Marsden
Hospital, London, UK.

M-T. Daniel
Institute de Recherches sur les
leucémies et les Maladies du Sang,
Hôpital Saint-Louis, Paris, France.

G. Flandrin
Institute de Recherches sur les
Leucémies et les Maladies du Sang,
Hôpital Saint-Louis, Paris, France.

D.A.G. Galton
Formerly MRC Leukaemia Unit, Royal
Postgraduate Medical School, London, UK.

H.R. Gralnick
Hematology Service, National Institutes
of Health, Bethesda, Maryland, USA.

C. Sultan
Service Central d'Hématologie-Immunologie,
Hôpital Henri Mondor, Creteil, France.

INDEX